Do No Harm

714X-DEFYING
A HOPELESS PROGNOSIS

The Scientific, Ethical, Legal and Spiritual
Revelation of Somatidian Orthobiology and 714X

Composed and Edited by
Charles Pixley and Caroline Ganz

with articles by:
Victor Pcnzer, MD, DMD, DSC.
Kenneth Brief
John W. Mattingly
William H. Moore, Jr., Esq.
Gaston Naessens
Victor Penzer, M.D., D.M.D., DSc.
Dictmar Schildwaechtcr, M.D., Ph.D.,
Otto Warburg, M.D.

et al.

Printed in the United States of America

Published by
Writers and Research, Incorporated

© 1992, continuing publications 2018, 2019

October 2019 Edition,
All Rights Reserved

Published by
Writers and Research. Incorporated

All articles contained herein are copyright protected. The information in this book is designed to provide accurate, authoritative information in regard to the subject matter covered. It is provided with the understanding that the publisher is not engaged in rendering medical or Segal services.

This office and its publication serve to synthesize and illumine the subject at hand. If you require medical or legal advice or the assistance of a licensed medical professional, the services of such a competent professional should be sought.

Library of Congress Cataloguing-in-Publication Data

Do no harm: the scientific, ethical, legal and spiritual revelation of somatidian orthobiology and 714X by Gaston Naessens, Dietmar Schildwaechter, William Moore, et al. p.c.

Includes bibliographies references and index.

1. Cancer-attemalive treatment. 2. Chronic diseases-Altemative treatment 3. Biological response modifiers-therapeutic use.

| Naessens, Gaston. || Schildwaechter, Dietmar. ||| Moore, William Harry, 1926- 1998

RC271.A62D6 1995

616.99"406—dc20   95-24978 CIP
ISBN 0964703-0-5

Table of Contents

HIPPOCRATIC OATH 3

HISTORY AND SOCIO-POLJTICS OF AMERICAN MEDICINE 25

BLOOD FEUD 37

QUESTIONS AND ANSWERS 79

READING THE BLOOD 86

714X A HIGHLY PROMSING NON-TOXIC TREATMENT FOR CANCER AND OTHER IMMINE DEFICIENCIES 89

General Purpose and Guidelines of this Research Protocol 105

PROTOCOL FOR USING 7 1 4 X 110

IMPORTANT DIETARY RECOMMENDATIONS 113

Lymphatic System 118

INJECTION TECHNIQUE 120

DeVilbiss AeroSonic™ Ultrasonic Nebulizer 122

THE PROTOCOL FOR THE USE OF AN ULTRASONIC NEBULIZER For SOMATO-THERAPY With 714X 124

Introducing the most highly calibrated Cancer-Profile and Immune-Spectrum Blood Test 127

Cancer and Immune Profile Test 130

Enzyme Therapy of Cancer by Max Wolf, M.D. 142

ENZYME THERAPY 155

Basic Notions in Microscopy 177

THE NAESSENS SOMATOSCOPE 181
THE DISCOVERY OF THE SOMATIC 182
THE NAESSENS ULTRAMICROSCOPE 183
THE PHYSIOLOGY OF BLOOD AS A TISSUE 188
CONCLUSION 231
ON THE PARASITIC THEORY OF CANCER 233
THE PRIME CAUSE AND PREVENTION OF CANCER 238
SCIENTIFIC INQUIRY, THE SOMATIDIAN THEORY and AIDS .264
Presented by Gaston Naessens 264
CONVENTIONAL OPTIONS 271
Cancer Chemotherapy 274
LEGAL REFERENCES 315
THE RIGHT TO TRY ACT 331
DETERMINATION 338

SPONSORS

Chief Medical Investigator and International Sponsor

Sovereign Consultants International. Ltd.

Dietmar Schildwaechter, M.D., Ph.D.

U.S. SPONSORS

Chief Medical Investigator and International Sponsor Sovereign Consultants International, Ltd. Dietmar Schildwaechter, M.D., Ph.D.

Chairman Institutional Review Board, IRB

Charles Pixley Writers and Research, Inc.

Charles Pixley

585-217-2191

"The care of human life and happiness and not its destruction is the first and only legitimate object of good government."

Thomas Jefferson

HIPPOCRATIC OATH

I call upon Apollo as healer, Asclepios, Hygeia and Panaceia, and all the gods and goddesses, making them my judges, that I will fulfill to the best of my power and discernment this oath and this accord;

that I will hold him who taught me this art as equal to my parents, that I will share his life, that I will share my resources with him when he is in need, that I will hold his progeny as equal to my brothers and teach them this art, if they ask to learn, without fee or contract, that I will share new instruction and lecture and all the remaining teachings with my sons and with the sons of my teacher and with students who have been bound by contract and oath of medical law, but with no other

I also will apply rules of life for the benefit of the sick according to my power and discernment to ward off harm and injustice.

I will not ever give a deadly drug, even if someone has asked for it, nor will I give instruction in this matter; likewise, I will not give abortive treatment to a woman; purely and according to the laws of nature will I oversee my life and my art

I will not use the knife, not even on those with stones, but will leave it to practitioners of this skill.

Into whatever houses I may go, I will enter for the benefit of the sick, being free from all willful injustice and any other destructive action, or seductive behavior towards the forms of women, free men or slaves.

Whatever I see or hear in the course of treatment or outside of treatment concerning the life of a patron, which must not be bruited about, I will not speak of, holding such things to be private.

While I fulfill my oath and do not violate it, may I reap the joys of life and art and be glorified by men for all time; should I fall short may the opposite be my fate.

translated by Caroline Grey Ganz

MATERIALIZING AN IMAGINATION

Mission Statement

Writers and Research, Inc.

Chronology

Conceived in 1990 as a synthesis of vision and practical application, Writers & Research, Inc. represents the expressed knowledge of select personalities whose works are, in our estimation, of benefit to the public. One such individual is Gaston Naessens who has created and discovered:

- an ULTRA High-powered microscope capable of viewing live matter at 30,000x.

- an indestructible pre-cursor to DNA in the blood.

- a means to pre-diagnose degenerative disease.

- a medicinal to stabilize the immune system in non-toxic treatment of degenerative disease.

- From **October 1990**, through **January of 1992** Charles Pixley appeared on approximately 100 local and national radio shows to alert the public to the existence of M. Naessens and Christopher Bird's book The Galileo of the Microscope.

- **January of 1992**, Writers and Research called the F.D.A. for information and subsequently founded what may be the only citizen formed Institutional Review Board (IRB) to present this knowledge and its uniform and correct application to the

American public and health care professionals and to provide a legally acceptable means to track the evolution of this investigation under the Code of Federal Regulations 21 part 56, known as Informed Consent. The F.D.A. officially added us to their list of IRBs after a formal inspection.

- **April 1992**, the first edition of the protocol <u>Do No Harm</u> was published to present this research and treatment as a basis upon which the inquiring patron can make an informed decision.

- **June 1992**, the IRB's Chief Medical Investigator, Dietmar Schildwaechter, M.D., Ph.D., former Congressman Berkely Bedell, who had used M. Naessens' 714X for metastatic cancer, and one co-investigator testified in person concerning this knowledge and treatment before the National Institutes of Health (NIH) hearings for the Office of Alternative Medicine. Writers and Research, Inc. presented written testimony for the record.

- **July 1992**, the F.D.A. published an import alert on 714X, banning its entry into the country.

- **March 1993**, we presented to Congress a general Health Care proposal pointing out that Universal Coverage means the availability of all aspects of health care offered globally and that managed competition is by definition an Anti-Trust violation.

- Late **March 1993**, our IRB was again inspected by a field agent of the FDA.

- **June 1993**, Writers & Research, Inc. registered with Congress as a lobbyist for truth.

- **August 1993**, Writers & Research President Charles Pixley was summoned by the F.D.A. to a meeting in Rockville, Maryland. He once again requested assistance of F.D.A. Officials in expediting the expensive, lengthy and risky approval process.

- **June 1994**, met with Governor Cuomo at NARTSH convention prior to Legislation passed in New York State granting Physicians freedom to practice any form of health care in the absence of harm to the patient without reprisal from medical or government agency.

- **June 1994**, met with Governor Wilson's Chief Economic Advisor in Sacramento, California, regarding health care policy in California.

- **July 1994**, the office of Writers and Research, Inc. was subject to a search and seizure by six federal agents who confiscated all private medical files without consent of the individuals, books and booklets, research materials on unrelated topics, all business files and records, stock certificates, rolodex and computers including modems, monitors, keyboards and software, because "they were used to print information on a substance that is banned in the United States."

- **August 1994**, Charles Pixley met with the Assistant Secretary for Health who oversees the FDA, CDC, NIH and Indian

Health Affairs to request and formal waiver to bypass the $250,000,000 standard approval process. **A claim of waiver was granted.**

- **September 1995**, met again with Governor Wilson's Staff in Sacramento, California, regarding victory over misuse of medical authority in a related legal battle in San Diego.
- **October 1995**, Charles Pixley was indicted on 19 counts of alleged "importation, distribution and conspiracy to distribute an unapproved medicine."

As of 1995, under this program thousands of patrons have petitioned for treatment with 714X and over 4,000 medical professionals have requested information concerning this research and treatment.

During this period of time the FDA continued to correspond with Mr. Pixley, as the Chairman of the Institutional Review Board of Writers and Research, Inc., as a Colleague.

This endeavor serves as a source of knowledge, data and empirical experience to be presented as evidence for the recognition and understanding of this research and its practical benefit.

Our modus operandi is to make available the protocol "Do No Harm" to ail those inquiring specifically about this treatment that they may make an informed decision based on all available options.

The origin of this project is with M. Naessens and dates back to the late 1940's. However, the scope of this enterprise is universal as knowledge knows no phenomenal boundaries.

The courage of conviction expressed by so many reminds us that limits are made to be transcended. Who recognize genius themselves have genius and can succeed in the restoration of ease in the place of disease in accordance with the laws of nature.

Medicine U.S.A, in the 1990s
by Dr. Victor Penzer
September 18, 1995

Many years ago, medicine appeared to be a noble profession. It was prior to W.W.H, before the concepts of genocide or ethnic cleansing became, despicable perhaps, but accepted acts of human civilization.

Medicine seemed to be the proper occupation for an idealist. The Hippocratic Oath 'Do No Harm" was taken seriously and generally heeded. Advertising by doctors was considered highly unethical

Times have changed and so have drastically the mores. Using humans as guinea pigs for medical experiments, with or without their knowledge and consent, goes on in many hospitals of high repute. Advertising by doctors, euphemistically ennobled to "marketing," is net only accepted but encouraged.

Advancements of medical technology brought new opportunities for plastic surgery, the original task of which was the repair of damaged parts of human anatomy and restoration of function. This degenerated mostly to become cosmetic surgery, catering to human vanity rather than to health.

Aggressive advertising offers alteration of human, nature-given sex organs, suggesting to gullible potential client's vague advantages, without ever mentioning any hazards. Truth, the whole truth and nothing but the truth is not the advertisers' Motto.

The "managed" or mismanaged, medical care gives doctors no time to diagnose or treat patients properly. The reports of biomedical laboratory tests guide doctors to prescribing from an arsenal of symptom-suppressing rather than health-restoring, expensive allopathic pharmaceuticals. In the process, these chemicals generate new ailments through insidious side- effects.

Naturopathic and homeopathic medicines are vilified by the disease industry under the pretense of protecting the public. Natural health practitioners are being harassed and persecuted. Health insurance, whether governmental or private, does not pay for alternate diagnostic or therapeutic intervention. The multi-billion-dollar disease-industry in feces legislators and law enforcement authorities. Functional Medicine, which offers diagnosis the pre-clinical stage or loss, is not being taught in medical school

Surgeons offer invasive treatments, even though surgery never removes the complete ailment, only a manifestation. Patients are rarely appraised of potential hazards. Thus, it is apparent that the Hippocratic Oath, "Do No Harm," must have been replaced by a hypocritic principle, "Tell No Truth."

Victor Penzer, MD, DMD, DSc, FASCD
Health Sciences Faculty, CIHS

Researchers, physicians and patrons whose interest, support and use of 714X research is notable:

Dr. Dietmar Schildwaechter, MD, PhD. former faculty member of the University of Pennsylvania School of Medicine.

Dr. Raymond Brown of New York City, a former Sloan-Kettering cancer researcher, told a pretrial press conference how he had treated one of his own patients with 714X for a pancreatic cancer that had proven resistant to all other forms of treatment. Naessens' therapy had prolonged the patient's life well over expectancy and kept him free of side effects, he said. Dr. Brown declared that while 714X was not a panacea, it deserved a place in the arsenal of weapons available to official medicine.

Dr. Florianne Pier, a Belgian physician "reported that over a four-month period, she had treated seven cancer patients with 714X. 'The product prolonged the lives, and eased the deaths, of two terminally afflicted patients,' she said, 'and has allowed the other five who came to me with seriously advanced cancerous states, to see every one of their symptoms disappear and to take up their lives as if they had never incurred the disease.'"

Dr. Daniel Perey, McMaster University Medical Center in Hamilton, Ontario, told the Canadian Government in 1972, "The scope and insight which Mr. Naessens has brought to this area of research potentially stand to benefit mankind and may be a source of pride for Canada."

Authorized copy found in <u>DO NO HARM</u>, according to the Saturday Night Magazine article, "Blood Feud," Dr. Perey was the original head of the investigation into Gaston Naessens' theories at McMaster University, a project funded by the Macdonald Stewart Foundation at the behest of David Stewart. Dr. Perey was later removed from direct involvement in the project, and the investigation apparently changed course due to the interests of a new research team with a different agenda.

Christopher Bird; author and friend of Gaston Naessens wrote: <u>The Persecution and Trial of Gaston Naessens.</u> Harvard graduate in Botonny and Peter Thompkins, co-authored <u>The Secret Life of Plants</u>, a WORLD WIDE and New York Times bestseller, Bird suffered a stroke at his home in Blairsville, GA, on 5/2/96 and died at the age of 68.

PATRON TESTIMONIALS

A close relative of George Bush, unidentified, Paul Wm. Roberts, reports:

In 1986, a woman who had been diagnosed with "one of the most devastating cancers: an oat-cell carcinoma of the lung that had metastasized to the brain, the adrenal gland, and the tissue between the lungs," according to her Doctor, Dietmar Schildwaechter, MD, PhD, recovered dramatically after being treated by Naessens 714X.

Schildwaechter did not find out that she was being treated by Naessens' until he began to inquire after monitoring dramatic improvements which he could not explain.

Mrs. Anne Vignal, wife of the former French Counsel General in Quebec.

"The most powerful argument for making Naessens treatment available is the example of people like Anne Vignal, wife of the former French Counsel General in Quebec, who went to medical doctors to find out why she had not conceived.

They told her infertility was due to a lethal form of leukemia and that she had only three to five years to live. Five years after being treated with 714X, she is very much alive and cancer-free--and the mother of a healthy son." Taken from "New Answer to Cancer," by Stephanie Hiller, Published in The Yoga Journal, but this link on the web no longer active.

Non-Hodgkin lymphoma Osteogenic Sarcoma

I started using 714X while undergoing treatment for a blood related cancer. I am certain that by using the product that it has been an important aspect for me to enter into remission and for feeling as healthy and strong as I do. Along with the traditional treatments I have received such as Chemotherapy and Rotuxin.

I feel that 714X has been an added benefit which has boosted my immune system. I have since completed two six-month maintenance treatments with the 714X and believe that it is a major factor in keeping me in remission and in building up my immune system. It is a product that I would recommend to anyone as being completely safe to use.

The staff at CERBE is always available to answer your questions and are truly honest and upfront and very trusting people. And as far as I am concerned that is the most important thing. The staff at CERBE has always made me feel like I am the first patient using their product and that they are truly concerned for my well-being. And that is special and very important when you are a cancer survivor. I am sure that you would feel the same way if you choose to use their product.

CAM

Blood cancer

Was diagnosed with atypical polycythemia rubra vera, a cancer of the blood, in 2002. This is a condition of too many red blood cells. The prescribed treatment is a phlebotomy when required. I had a phlebotomy in February, March and April of this year.

In early May, I began 714X, and for the next three months my blood was normal. I also made lifestyle changes and am taking supplements. I required a phlebotomy in August and October buy my blood work was normal again in November. My next blood test will be the end of December.

I am most heartened by this obvious success. It is only a very short time that I have been on 714X, roughly seven months, and already indications are that things are progressing on 714X, roughly seven months, and already indications are that things are progressing well.

My energy level is noticeably improved and I am sleeping better than I have in years. My blood pressure, which has been high for 20 years, is also very much improved. I am grateful for the availability of 714X and look forward to using it for the continued improvement of my health.

A. W. Canada

Neuroectodermal tumor

I was diagnosed with Primitive Neuroectodermal tumor in 1985 at the age of 13. It started in the nasal passage. Surgery was done and within a few months it grew back, had filled the right sinuses and was pushing to get into the brain. Again, surgery was done, then radiation and about 2 yrs of chemo. Finished chemo August 1987. My mother passed away October 1987 with colon cancer. Then, in 1991 it came back and in the right kidney. That kidney was removed. Then in 1993, it came back in the left lower lobe lung.

Surgery and then a year of chemo. This was worse than the first time I did it. Within a few months of finishing chemo, it was back in the right lower lobe. Surgery was done - 6 days before my nursing graduation. I was told that they could take out my bone marrow, do full body radiation, and a onetime dose of melphalan which is a mustard gas. This would give 30% remission. No "cure".

I would have a 10% chance of dying from the procedure, have a chance of coming out with aplastic anemia and would be in the hospital for 2-3 months (part of that in total isolation). I had the Doctors provide me studies of their proposed treatment. Everyone died according to the studies. I found out about 714X from my step-mom's brother. I started the treatment and 3 months after my last surgery, I got married, bought a house and passed my nursing state boards. I felt GOOD!!!

I am going to be 14 yrs. cancer free. I have received my second-degree black belt in karate and am currently a nurse for hospice. I tell my patients about the 714X although none have opted to do it. I think most of these people have been put in such a state of depression because of the "terminal" news and because of some of the harsh treatments they have just finished. I truly believe that God has designed our bodies to heal themselves, they just need the right things in them, that's all. Anyway, I want to thank you again for what you guys are doing!

JC, KS, USA

Lupus and Cytomeglo Virus

My name is L.E, I am 40 years old women. I have been ill for a number of years with Cytomeglo Virus and later Lupus. I tested positive in 1985 and have dealt with it mentally and with cortisone treatment.

In 1999 I fell very ill while working for a large farming enterprise. Stress, long hours, exhaustion all added to this. After numerous tests I tested positive for Lupus. So bad that the specialists suggested chemotherapy etc., which I turned down immediately. I phoned a very good friend in the medical world who put me onto Gus Stevens.

Gus suggested that I start a course of 714X injections that came from Canada as he had had remarkable results with his son with cancer. Lupus is a degenerative viral disease and the injections were specifically for this. I started immediately. I was very ill at this stage, with no energy, chest pains that I could barely breath and basically bed ridden.

I knew that 714X would not work immediately and that it was going to take time, so I was very patient. Injecting every evening at the same time, eating a corrective diet and rest all helped.

After two treatments I started feeling better and by the end of four treatments I was as fit as a fiddle. Back to the normal old self and normal daily work. I do have to be careful of getting stressed and over working. In July 2001 I did get ill again but not as bad as before so I immediately started another course and after two courses, I was back on track again.

Lupus will never be cured. It is put into remission. I did test negative for Lupus after all my treatment, so let's hope it stays that way. I was told that it would not treat CMV but to my surprise it put it into remission and have not had a touch of any symptoms since, even though my blood tests did come back positive for the CMV.

As of today, I am healthier than ever.

Bladder tumor

The symptoms began in June of 2007 (primarily bleeding and clots in the urine) and an ultrasound determined there was a bladder tumor. As our primary care physician was a Naturopathic MD and my husband was completely philosophically opposed to an allopathic approach and treatment, we decided to work with her and jointly approach a healing process. Fairly early on, our ND suggested 714X as a possibility in my husband's treatment regimen and loaned us the Video to watch, but we were hesitant initially, not understanding quite how it all worked and - at this stage - not quite sure what we were up against with the cancer diagnosis. So, we worked with a lot of different treatment modalities with our ND, and succeeded in slowing the growth of the tumor, but it did slowly increase in size. It was a delicate balance to address the underlying infection and toxins we were certain were at the root of the problem, prevent the tumor from growing too quickly while we addressed that underlying issue, and keeping the bleeding under control. An episode of rapid and fairly sudden blood loss in August of 2008 required an Emergency Room visit and overnight hospital stay to administer a transfusion of 4 units of blood. After this, treatment with our ND continued, as well as other changes we knew in our hearts and minds were necessary in our lives, if healing was to be achieved.

Fast-forward to May of 2010 - a relatively long period of mild to moderate to severe blood loss left my husband weak and very debilitated, so we wound up in the Emergency Room again. This time, he'd reached a point where the medical personnel were concerned about the strain the blood loss was having on his heart and he was admitted to the ICU. The blood transfusions were begun almost immediately. The CT scan done there showed the tumor that we knew was there, but only one (a previous scan had indicated there was another, smaller one on the bladder wall, as well) - it was blocking the right kidney ureter.

They recommended flushing the bladder to clear out the clots, doing a cystoscopy, and, whilst there, surgically removing the tumor basically by cauterizing it (no cutting). Weak, a little "fogbound" and a little overwhelmed, my husband initially was not in favor of the procedure, but we gave it a lot of thought overnight and by morning consented. The Urologist was not sure he could remove the entire tumor, as it was large enough to stretch the limits of this procedure. It's difficult to describe the relief that washed over me when the Urologist told me he "got it all" - another step of hope forward. Unfortunately, the oncology report indicated the cancer had penetrated the bladder wall - it was in the muscle tissue. A stent was left in place to the right ureter. Two nights in the ICU, one night in a regular room, loads of flushing, one surgery and 6 units of blood later, we went home.

Just before this trip to the hospital, we had determined we needed to try the 714X as our ND recommended, and had ordered it. We started it as soon as it arrived in the mail about a week after being released from the hospital. A short time after the hospital stay, we had a consultation with the Urologist and his prognosis was not good - in fact, it was pretty depressing. He recommended a removal of the bladder and prostate and a "bag". He said that there was a 50% chance that the cancer had already metastasized to somewhere else in the body.

It was the only "treatment" the Urologist suggested and my husband declined it. The Urologist said he would monitor the progress and recommended another cystoscopy and removal of the stent 3 months later - in August. It wound up being the same day as the end of Round 4 of 714X. The cystoscopy showed some spots that the Urologist identified as being cancer-related; he said this was what he expected, although he thought he'd find more of those "spots" than he did. Kidney function, thankfully, was basically back to normal. The Urologist suggested another cystoscopy in 3 months - in November - one day into Round 9.

At this time, he could find only one tiny tumor, which he removed immediately using the cauterization technique he'd used with such success in the hospital - this time in his office. He took a long time looking around with the scope and was amazed that there was no other evidence of the cancer to be seen in the bladder. He said he couldn't believe it was the same bladder he was looking at and even went so far as to say things like, "Once in a career does one see something like this!" (oddly, his notes do not express this exuberant surprise). The oncology report determined it was the same type of cancer, but this time had not penetrated the bladder wall. We were very happy with the results and cautiously optimistic about the progress.

As recommended, we returned again in February - and to our delight and the Urologist's continued surprise, there was only scarring on the bladder wall from the surgery and no other evidence of the cancer visible in the cystoscopy. He told us to keep doing whatever we're doing and to come back in 3-4 months. After completing 10 Rounds of 714X, my husband took a short break, but resumed with the 3 recommended consecutive Rounds at the end of April. Several days into Round 2 of those 3, my husband had another cystoscopy; this time a tiny, 6 mm papillary tumor was discovered on the opposite side to the original mass on the bladder wall, which he again removed with the "Bugbee".

While we were obviously hoping for another totally clear report, the urologist was actually very encouraging and said we had, in a way, come full circle and if all we were going to see was these small but high-grade recurrences, he could now recommend conventional treatment options - BCG (introducing a form of the tuberculosis bacteria into the bladder to kill off cancer cells) and suggested in his report that there was a small chance that my husband had been cured by the resection!

There is no question in our minds that 714X has been an essential component of the healing progress my husband has made thus far and we are hopeful of a full recovery with no recurrences. We plan to continue with some form of 714X regimen and to continue with the regular cystoscopy monitoring of the bladder.

Leukemia

I was fighting acute leukemia 18 years ago and Gaston Naessens not only selflessly helped save my life but also saved my leg from being amputated. I just wanted to write a quick message THANKING him and everyone there who care so much for others!

With admiration,

EC

Ovarian cancer

I was diagnosed with stage 3 Ovarian Cancer 8 years ago. I was re-diagnosed 3 years ago with metastasis Ovarian Cancer in my colon and liver. My doctor didn't give me much hope for survival.
I heard about 714X through a friend who had used it when she was diagnosed with Breast Cancer at the early age of 29. She is still alive 12 years later. I had surgery for the removal of the tumor in my colon. However, nothing could be done about my liver at that time. So, I decided to try 714X. I had nothing to lose. I tried 714X. My doctor then sent me for a CT-Scan and I no longer had any cancer in my liver. I have continued to use 714X and I am now cancer free, and have been for three years.
I can't say enough about the product and the people I deal with to obtain it. 714X has given me my life back. »
C. P. New Hampshire, USA

Breast cancer

I was under the treatment of an oncologist after I was told I had breast cancer in 1999. I had chemo followed by a mastectomy and then radiation. I continued seeing the doctor and having checkups. After two years, I wasn't feeling good and insisted on a mammogram on my existing breast. After the results were returned, they noticed some lumps on my lungs and decided to do a cat scan. That showed the cancer was also in my liver.

A friend of a friend told me that she had used 714X and that I should try it. "Never" I said... my oncologist tells me what I should do. Well, after thinking it over and seeing that my cancer was quickly spreading with the traditional treatment, I said I would try it. The nurse at the oncology center told me about a woman that was giving her father the injections. I called her and she showed me how to inject myself.

From that day forward I have been using 714X. My CEA level the tumor marker was 8, 6 in February 2003. After being on 714X it is now gone!

Anything below 3 is normal! I have had two cat scans, one in September 2003 and one in December 2003. They have both come back as being stable with some shrinkage. My oncologist cannot believe it. Would I choose to give myself a shot each morning to remain healthy as opposed to doing chemo and becoming violently sick? Absolutely, any time!

I was once skeptical and now am a true believer. My whole attitude is more positive because I can now see the results of 714X and that makes me fight harder. I wish I could have everyone with cancer aware of this product. I'm sure there would be a lot fewer deaths.

I cannot say enough about 714X and lonely hope that eventually everyone will be using it to fight this dreaded disease.

Karen Christo, MA

HISTORY AND SOCIO-POLJTICS OF AMERICAN MEDICINE

Synopsized from several articles

by William H. Moore, Jr., Esq., Attorney-at-Law, Hom.MD

The Beginning

Science is knowledge (Latin scio, I know). Modern science was cast in its present mold in the seventeenth century by Descartes and Newton who assumed that reality was limited to phenomena accessible to the five senses, materially quantifiable, that each effect is the product of a single cause and that the whole is the sum of the parts.

These basic assumptions are generally accepted as truth although the theory of relativity of time, energy and matter and the observations of quantum mechanics indicate otherwise.

The history of medicine begins with the Aryan migration to the sub-continent of India at some time not readily identifiable by modern anthropology or history. The knowledge held by this ancient culture was orally transmitted until written down as the body of works known as the Vedas.

Ayurveda, part of the fourth and youngest Veda, concerns itself with physical health and reveals the cause of disease as ignorance, the cure knowledge, it describes in detail the nature, function and interaction of the three planes of existence—body, life and mind—the conditions resulting from refraction of the original order and the appropriate treatments thereof.

All ancient forms of medicine contain some aspects of Ayurveda, increasingly obscured in ritual and dogma as they involve through time until a complete lack of the original understanding gives way to an analytical form of material knowledge aspiring for objective reality.

In the early 18th Century the healing arts were comprised of three separate and competing schools: the solidist school, represented by William Cullen, John Brown, and Benjamin Rush, also known as the regular, orthodox or allopathic school; the homeopathic school founded by Samuel Hahnemann; and the eclectic school comprising native herbal practitioners and the trained physicians who recognized and espoused their botanical knowledge--the latter two groups becoming united in competition with allopathy.

The two groups were opposed from the outset in their underlying philosophies or approaches to the nature and acquisition of knowledge. Both schools acknowledged investigation through the senses to determine the-phenomenal reality.

The adherents of the allopathic school then proceeded through deductive reasoning or by analogy with other sciences-physics, mechanics, hydraulics, chemistry-to ascertain and conclude what they could not see of the inner workings of the human body.

The homeopathic school held that the inner workings of the body were not accessible to understanding as they were not analogous to any other science, had their own laws and the state of disease was non-material.

The shortcomings of both schools were reflected in each other-the materialist limitations of allopathy mirrored the agnostic conclusions of homeopathy.

Rival medical organizations were created in the 1840's representing the two schools of thought and practice, competing for supremacy in the market place of medical enterprise. The history of this hostility wends its way through politics and economics, as must every human endeavor.

The conflict of ideology and its result is summed up by American Philosophy William James in an address to the Massachusetts state legislature in 1898:

"In spite of the rival schools appealing to experience, their conflict is much more like that of two philosophers or two theologies. Tour experience, says one side to the other, simply isn't fit to count."

During the end of the 19th Century the health care industry received an enormous financial infusion from the Rockefeller and Carnegie fortunes. John D. Rockefeller wished to establish a medical institute at the University of Chicago that was neither allopath nor homeopath, but simply scientific in its investigations into medical science." This was not to happen.

The director of the Rockefeller Institute had close ties to allopathic medicine and Rockefeller was persuaded to abandon his dream of scientific synthesis. Until his death, however, he retained a homeopathic physician for his personal health care.

In the 1920's, the school of allopathy was legally invested by the Medical Practices Acts, passed by most State Legislatures, making it, by tacit agreement, the only legally practicable and thus bona fide healing art.

State and Federal Regulation

In the last quarter of the nineteenth century the move towards medical licensure was initiated by the American Medical Association, the Trade Association for the Allopathic School.

When the process was begun, State Legislatures typically created three separate State Boards of Medical examiners, to examine and license medical practitioners of the Allopathic, Homeopathic and Eclectic Schools of Medical Practice; in many states the Osteopathic School was also given a Board of Examiners.

Shortly thereafter, other health care practitioners were also given licenses which carried out certain exceptions to the universal licensure of physicians, such as Dentists, Podiatrists, Pharmacists, Nurses, Midwives, Physiotherapists and eventually, Acupuncturists.

The licenses granted to these practitioners were to treat any human disease, disorder or condition by drugs, surgery or any other means and all persons not so licensed were forbidden to undertake such activities for compensation.

There is a National Federation of State Boards of Medical Examiners which attempts to set over-all policy for State Licensing Boards and this is a private not a governmental organization.

There is universal licensure of physicians and surgeons, osteopathic physicians and surgeons, dentists, chiropractic physicians and there is considerable variation as to the licensure of Naturopathic physicians and Oriental medical practitioners (acupuncturists) on a state by state basis.

Despite the state by state variation, allot these practitioners practice in a virtually uniform fashion, all have trade associations and specialty societies which are national in scope and all receive fairly standardized training.

The Food and Drug Administration was created in 1938 as a federal agency to ensure that food, drugs and cosmetics moving in interstate commerce were unadulterated, contained what was stated on the label and were thereby safe for human consumption.

The scope of this agency was strengthened in 1962 with the Kefauffer Amendments to that Act which contained an efficacy requirement and gave the FDA far more power to control both drugs and information about drugs.

The agency has lawful jurisdiction over some Foods, Drugs and medical devices which are in interstate commerce and has no jurisdiction over the practice of medicine or other healing professions.

Despite this rather clear distinction, the agency now uses its enforcement powers and state regulatory agencies to interfere with the practice of non-allopathic health care and suppress the use of techniques of healing and of products which are outside its regulatory jurisdiction.

These circumstances have fostered a standardized system of American Health Care which is unable to:

1) Control the resurgence of Tuberculosis in the country;
2) Control the rising rate of Cancer deaths;
3) Control the rising rate of coronary artery deaths;
4) Lower the infant mortality rate;
5) Find an effective treatment for AIDS.

There are answers to all these deficiencies and many of them lie outside the scope of allopathic practice.

The Federal Act was not intended to give the agency any control over the practice of medicine or other health care professions and both its language and many decisions of Federal Courts make that clear.

Anti-Trust Actions against the A.M.A.

The Federal Trade Commission brought an enforcement action against the AMA and its component societies resulting in information concerning anti-competitive misconduct. Subsequently a private enforcement action by four chiropractors resulted in further permanent injunctions against anti-competitive misconduct.

The latter action, *Wilk, et al. v. A.M.A.* was based upon a campaign conducted by the

A.M.A. through its Department of Investigation and Council Against Quackery "to first contain then eliminate Chiropractic."

During the litigation, the Department of Investigation and the Council Against Quackery were hurriedly disbanded by the A.M.A. and files of these organizations were handed over to a private organization, the National Council against Health Care Fraud, NCAHF, which, funded by the Pharmaceutical Advertising Council and working in conjunction with the F.D.A., continues the anti-competitive campaigns as a private organization.

The AMA initially formed a sub rosa organization, the "Health Information Control Council" which included members from several bureaucratic regulatory agencies. This was also broken up during the Wilk litigation.

As a part of the Wilk litigation, the Court held that calling a licensed competitor a Quack would constitute an antitrust offense. Since that time the NCAHCF has substituted the word "fraud" for "quack" in its anti-competitive campaigns which increasingly utilize State and Federal agents as instruments of prosecution.

This combination has already threatened the availability and quality of goods and services and astronomically increased their price in the medical market place.

The Food and Drug Administration, created to perform some proper regulatory functions, is devoting many of its resources to illegal functions not contained in its enabling legislation, in direct violation of the clearly articulated policies of the States and not permissible under the Constitution.

Our responsibility is to determine the course of action to bring this agency under control that it may comport itself in accordance with the intent of Congress representing the will of the people.

The Legal and Ethical Foundation

Freedom of choice in matters of opinion and personal property is a fundamental constitutional right.

In **1943**, Justices Black, Douglas and Murphy wrote, "If there is any fixed star in our constellation it is that no official, high or petty, can prescribe what shall be orthodox in politics, nationalism, religion, or other matters of opinion or force Citizens to confess by word or act their faith therein.

"The right to be let alone is indeed the beginning of all freedom. Part of our claim to privacy is in the prohibiting of the Fourth Amendment against unreasonable searches and seizures. It gives the guarantee that a man's home is his castle beyond invasion either by inquisitive or by officious people....

"He may not be compelled against his will to attend a religious service; he may not be forced to make affirmation or observe a ritual that violates his scruples; he may not be made to accept one religious, political, or philosophical creed against another.

"Freedom of religion and freedom of speech guaranteed by the First Amendment give more than the privilege to worship, to write, to speak as one chooses; they give freedom not to do or act as the government chooses. West Virginia State Board of Education v. Barnett, 319 U.S. 624, 634, 639, (1943).

The Supreme Court declared in 1943: "One's right to life, liberty and property... and other fundamental rights may not be submitted to a vote; they depend on the outcome of no election." Ibid.

"The First Amendment in its respect for the conscience of the individual honors the sanctity of thought and belief. To think as one chooses, to believe what one wishes are important aspects of the Constitutional right to be let alone." Justice Douglas dissenting, Public *Utilities Commission v. Pollak*, 343 U.S. 451 (1952).

The following material Is excerpted from
"Patients' Rights to Receive Unorthodox Cancer Treatments in the United States"

by Kenneth A. Brief

The "Frye Rule"

In 1923 A Federal Appeals court ruled that the lawyers for a convicted murderer named Frye couldn't present the results of a "systolic blood pressure test," an earlier version of the lie detector test, because it had not won "general acceptance in the particular field in which it belongs." Since then federal judges have adopted the "Frye rule" as the standard for admissibility of scientific evidence.

The issues implicated by patients' rights to unorthodox treatments go as deep as any imaginable. They involve fundamental rights, freedoms and liberties held sacred in the Constitution. They pertain to life and death decisions of the most intimate and excruciating kind.

The legal struggle over cancer patient's rights to unorthodox treatments results from an unresolved conflict in our law: a person's fundamental right to free choice interpreted from the Bill of Rights as the right of privacy versus government's obligation to protect us under the health and welfare clause of the Constitution.

Strict informed consent regulations would be an effective way to protect patients using experimental or unorthodox treatments, especially when viable orthodox treatment options exist. This is a way to preserve patients' freedom to choose, satisfy the government's duty to protect as well as safeguard physicians from malpractice liability.

It is simply unscientific for orthodox medical practitioners to persist in overlooking medical evidence in any form, suggesting new ways of healing cancer.

The growing awareness of the grave limitations of many orthodox cancer treatments, may be the reason the Court of Appeals made a very significant ruling for cancer patients seeking the right to receive unorthodox treatments. This is the case Schneider v. Revici 817F.2d.987 (2nd Cir, 1987).

The heart of this case is the ruling on assumption of risk, ibid 990. By applying assumption of risk to a medical malpractice action, patients acquire a new legal right to receive non-conventional treatments because they bear the responsibility of their choice.

'While a patient should be encouraged to exercise care for his own safety, we believe that an informed decision to avoid surgery and conventional chemotherapy is within the patient's right to determine what shall be done with his own body. Schloendorff v. Society of the New York Hospital, 211 N.Y. 125, 129, 105 N.E. 92 (1914). Schneider at 994.

Doctors in this country are determined to be using appropriate medical procedures based on two similar legal doctrines, depending on the state in which they practice. They are the "deviation from accepted practice" and the "reasonably prudent practitioner" standard.

The Court of Appeals is saying that an unorthodox cancer practice, which by definition would be considered malpractice, still maybe effective treatment. Traditionally, this would be a contradiction in terms but this decision clearly says it is not.

Justice Brandeis in his famous dissent in the Olmstead case wrote:

"The makers of our Constitution undertook to secure conditions favorable to the pursuit of happiness. They recognized the significance of man's spiritual nature, of his feelings and of his intellect.

"They knew that only a part of the pain, pleasure and satisfactions of life are to be found in material things. They sought to protect Americans in their beliefs, their thoughts, their emotions and their sensations.

"They conferred, as against the Government, the right to be let alone - the most comprehensive of rights and the right most valued by civilized men. To protect that right, every unjustifiable intrusion by the Government upon the privacy of the individual, whatever the means employed, must be deemed a violation…

"Experience should teach us to be most on our guard to protect liberty when the Government's purposes are beneficent. Men born to freedom are naturally alert to repel invasion of their liberty by evil minded rulers. The greatest dangers to liberty lurk in insidious encroachment by men of zeal, well-meaning but without understanding."

<u>Olmstead v. United States</u> 277 U.S. 438, 478, 479 (1927)

BLOOD FEUD
by Paul William Roberts

Gaston Naessens claims to have discovered a new way of looking at blood that could revolutionize the treatment of cancer. Why does the Medical establishment consider him so dangerous?

In 1939, a French-born biologist named Gaston Naessens was arrested in Quebec and charged with four counts of illegal practice of medicine and one count of contributing to the death of a patient.

The patient, a woman with metastasized breast cancer in the terminal stages, had refused all conventional treatments and insisted instead on taking a camphor-based medicinal that Naessens had developed.

The medicinal, which he called 714X, was designed not to destroy cancer cells in the way of conventional treatments but to bolster the immune system and help the body heal itself.

Naessens, who had a tiny private lab on the banks of the Magog River in the Eastern Townships, had instructed a close friend of the woman's in how to inject the substance into the lymphatic node in the groin. She received injections for seven months before she died in July, 1984.

The prosecution wished to prove that Naessens' patient might have stood a chance if she had pursued conventional treatment. The corollary was proving that Naessens knew his alternative treatment to be worthless--that he was a charlatan hoping to profit from the desperation of someone in the throes of terminal illness.

The prosecution was not fooling around-the charge of contributing to the woman's death carried a potential life sentence.

The trial, which made the front pages of Quebec newspapers for three weeks in November, 1989, opened with a parade of doctors and scientists testifying to the scientific untenability of 714X and the spurious nature of Naessens' theories of cancer and its treatment.

In the media, a sketchy, negative image of the man began to emerge; he claimed to have invented a microscope that could reveal the mysteries of living blood. He claimed to have discovered, through his studies of blood, something he called a somatid, which he said was a precursor of DNA and the absolute ground zero of life.

He claimed to have identified a sixteen-stage cycle through which the somatid passed, and claimed that he could link the various phases of that cycle with the health (or ill health) of a patient.

He'd drawn the ire of medical authorities in his homeland; he'd been forced out of France twenty-five years earlier. He'd set up in the quiet backwater of Quebec, his critics said, hoping to evade medical scrutiny.

By the time the defense was ready to present its case to the jury, the mood was grim in the Naessens camp. But it soon changed. Witness after witness took the stand to describe the horrors of their battles with cancer and the apparent cures they'd finally achieved after using Naessens' treatment.

Gerald Godin, politician, journalist, poet testifying on the biologist's behalf, outlined his struggle with a brain tumor that he believed 714X had helped to check. The French ambassador to the Seychelles told a similar story.

in the courtroom the gratitude to Naessens was so apparent and emotions running so high that the prosecutor chose not to cross-examine defense witnesses on "Human grounds."

Moreover, the testimonials to Naessens' integrity were overwhelming: He'd never promised a cure, never told one of them to discontinue conventional treatment, and never asked for payment.

When Gilles Vigneault, chansonnier and bard, a Quebecois folk hero, arrived from Paris to show his support for Naessens, the effect was electrifying. To the press during a court lunch break, Vigneault described what was happening to Naessens as a "witch hunt" and went on to sing the praises of alternative medicine.

He concluded: "One must seek, on humanity's behalf, medical progress unblocked by pharmaceutical lobbyism that, together with that of arms mongers, is one of the world's most powerful."

The jury was not long in coming to a verdict: Acquittal on all five counts. The Journal de Montreal went to town, its front page headlined NAESSENS ACQUITTED.

A sidebar, however, bore the headline "It's Twenty-Five Years Now That This Farce Has Continued," quoting Dr. Augustin Roy, the head of the Quebec Medical Corporation, the professional self-regulating and licensing body that had pushed for charges to be laid against Naessens.

The Trial, Roy said, was "wholly incomplete"; the prosecutor should have "savagely cross-examined every one of the patients who had testified on Naessens' behalf....

"All the patients who testified simply don't know the difference between feeling healthy and being healthy... All of them should stand at attention or, more properly, get down on their knees to thank orthodox medicine for having kept them alive."

Roy apparently had not noticed that the majority of Naessens' patients were refugees from conventional medicine, which had either written them off or offered a treatment that frequently seemed worse than the disease.

And Roy was not about to relent. Within weeks of the not-guilty verdict, eighty-two more counts of practicing medicine without a license were brought against Naessens, each carrying the threat of a $35,000 fine.

As was clear from this rhetoric, Augustin Roy wasn't fighting any more to protect innocent patients from an unscrupulous quack. He was fighting to protect his profession from an alternative vision of healing, an alternative model of disease processes, and a press that kept on insisting that this heretic, Gaston Naessens, was the Galileo of modern medicine and the microscope.

Naessens himself prefers a comparison with Antoine Bechamp. Not so well known as Galileo and not so persecuted for his "heresies," Bechamp, a professor of biochemistry and dean of the Faculty of Medicine at the University of Lilies, France, in the last decades of the nineteenth century, had been Louis Pasteur's major adversary.

The controversy between Pasteur and Bechamp--now a forgotten episode in medical history-had been the scientific equivalent of front-page news and concerned the very nature of disease itself.

Bechamp believed that the cause of disease lay within the entire system of the body; Pasteur insisted that disease came from without, which fitted with the formulation of his now famous and standard germ theory. It seems likely that both men were right to a certain degree, but Pasteur was a tireless self-promoter while Bechamp was diffident and somewhat reclusive.

Pasteur's model was also more appealing to physicians who wanted a definite disease target on which they could make war, rather than a state of good health they had to delicately maintain. Thus: the Pasteur Institute, on the one hand, and on the other, a baffled shrug from most doctors if Bechamp's name comes up.

Under his microscope more than a century ago, Bechamp had observed in fermenting solutions tiny particles, which he called microzymas, that appeared to have powerful catalytic effects—

facilitating change while remaining essentially unchanged themselves.

He went on to note the presence of these particles in the bodies of animals, coming to the conclusion not only that they were the most fundamental form of all living matter but that they were essential to any form of life, from cell division and basic bacteria up.

What seemed most extraordinary to Bechamp was the observation that the microzymas could apparently actively participate in the destruction of an organism without being destroyed themselves.

Indeed, their indestructibility was such that he believed a French paleontologist had found evidence of them in 60-million-year-old limestone from the early Cenozoic era, the period when mammals first started to develop on earth.

How Naessens became Bechamp's inheritor is a bit of a convoluted story. The youngest child of a banker, Naessens was born in 1924 in Roubaix, near Lille in northern France. As a child he showed a mechanical proclivity that both amazed and terrified his parents. From manipulating Meccano sets at five the boy went on to build his own motorcycle and then an airplane just big enough to carry him—which his mother burned before it could take its maiden flight.

The Second World War broke out as Naessens was beginning to study physics, chemistry, and biology at the University of Lille. When the Nazis occupied the city both he and his professors ended up in exile near Nice, where he continued his studies towards a degree.

Naessens received a diploma from the Union Scientifique Nationale Francaise, the semi- official institution that operated during the chaotic conditions of the war. But in what turned out to be a typically independent fashion he never bothered to ask for the formal equivalencies the de Gaulle government issued after the war. Consequently, he's been accused of having no academic credentials.

The young man went to work in a laboratory for blood analysis, and hated both the routine job and the imprecision of the microscopes he used. Blurrily he was able to observe something in the blood that had so far not been defined: other researchers had seen it, too, and called it "dross in the blood."

He needed a better instrument. Searching the literature for research on blood and microscopy, Naessens learned of a nineteenth century French biologist now best known as the

"noon lunatic." Emile Doyen claimed to have observed, through an ordinary microscope, particles in human blood that were visible only around noon during the months of May and June' Naessens was as willing to laugh at the notion as anyone, but began to wonder whether there was any scientific explanation of Doyen's findings.

There was: During May and June, in the south of France and at around noon, the natural light available to anyone using a microscope contained far more ultraviolet light than at any other time of the year.

The work of the noon lunatic became the basis for the microscope Naessens went on to develop in the late 1940s, working in a lab funded by his mother at the family home in Lyon.

An extreme and as yet un-duplicated version of what is now called phase or dark-field microscopy, Naessens' instrument allowed him to examine living blood not only at high magnifications but with extremely high resolution.

Although an electron microscope can approach 400,000 X magnification, it can do so only with fixed and dead tissue. Naessens' microscope, which identified particles with light refraction rather than staining, could approach 30,000 X with living tissue at a resolution of 150 angstroms (one angstrom is one-hundred-millionth of a centimeter)

The uniqueness of the microscope has to do with the way Naessens manipulates the light source to achieve that extraordinary resolution. (Several optical companies have approached him over the years but Naessens has been unwilling to give over control of his life's work to big manufacturers.)

What the tool unlocked for Naessens the researcher was a deep view- the deepest and as yet unsurpassed view-into the processes of living blood.

Naessens started by looking at preparations of his own blood- pricking his finger, transferring the drop to a slide, watching until the fresh blood began to clot.

Through his microscope, he observed what he maintains are Bechamp's microzymas: the most fundamental particles of living matter that exist. He called them somatids (tiny bodies) and through seven years of observation concluded that they appeared to play an extraordinary role.

No cell division was possible without (hem; they were seemingly a precursor to DNA, and probably the bridge between energy and matter. He found them all but indestructible, surviving carbonization temperatures of more than 200 degrees C and 50,000 REMs of radiation (more than enough to kill a person); they were also unaffected by chemical agents.

With a better tool to use, Naessens could go way beyond Bechamp, who was able to see only the largest of these microzymas. Naessens observed the somatid in human and animal blood to develop in a form-changing cycle.

The first three changes of this cycle-somatid, spore, and double spore—were apparently not only normal in healthy organisms but crucial to their existence in that no cell division could take place without them. Having studied what he took to be healthy blood, he began to study blood from people he knew to be diseased, referred to him by physicians. Unhealthy blood looked drastically different, and exhibited somatids in not a three-stage but a sixteen-stage cycle.

The other thirteen stages were apparently the result of an immune system under stress, and seemed to signal the likelihood of degenerative disease up to two years before any symptoms appeared in the organism.

Naessens began to believe that with observation of the somatid cycle-in effect, monitoring the physiology of blood-he could figure out when it was possible to intervene to prevent illness.

Take cancer, for instance. Every body every day produces a few cancer cells and a normal immune system destroys them. But when that system comes under stress, its ability to fight is impaired and the cancer cells proliferate.

When the ovum is fertilized by a sperm, growth (or cell division) begins: two, four, eight, and so on. There are many such divisions before cells begin to specialized, some becoming skin, some liver, some heart, and so on.

This specialization is controlled by a series of growth hormones that "talk" to the various cells' nuclei. These intracellular commands come from various sources-lymphocytes, for example, controlled by one, liver cells by another.

In normal circumstances, the growth hormones are controlled by inhibitors in the blood, but when a system is stressed these inhibitors diminish and more growth hormones are liberated.

The result is almost a reversal of the cells' "education," They return to a simpler state, losing their individuality and "remembering" only basic functions from their origins, chief of which is the ability to multiply rapidly and chaotically.

This, it is thought, is malignancy, the pathological cells resembling primitive organisms that have forgotten everything they have learned.

Naessens, through the microscope he called a "somatoscope," was able to observe the consequences of the diminution of sanguine inhibitors and the liberation of the growth hormone by watching the three-stage somatid cycle in the blood suddenly proceeding on through its full sixteen polymorphic stages-before patients had any conventionally diagnosable sign that they were ill.

His next challenge was to figure out how to bolster the immune system to correct the imbalances in the body that led to disease. He began experimenting with ways to combat the effects of degenerative or cancerous cells by neutralizing their mode of replication- developing a series of novel anticancer products.

These early medicinals proved effective enough over a fourteen-year period for Swiss and German pharmacies to put them on sale and for numerous doctors to administer them to patients. (By 1964, more than 10,000 people had been treated.)

On the strength of his sales, Naessens was able to move his lab to Paris in the mid-'50s. But in Paris he came to the attention of French medical authorities, after complaints from some pharmacists and physicians that this un-credentialed young biologist was dabbling in healing.

In the early 1960s, Naessens was twice brought before the bar. He was fined heavily, his Paris laboratory sealed and much of his equipment confiscated.

He tried to start again on the island of Corsica, but Corsica was still France. Patients began again to seek him out and the authorities were soon after him. Naessens decided that he had to pursue his work far from France, in a place he believed to be more open-minded. He left Corsica for Canada in 1964, carrying only a few key components of his microscope with him.

Unable to obtain any funding to pursue his research, Naessens began life as an immigrant by working days in an electronics repair shop in Oka, Quebec. The nights and the weekends were reserved for refining his somatoscope. Through some work he did repairing scientific equipment for several Quebec Universities, he got what seemed to be his first break.

A senior professor at the University of Sherbrooke hired him as a consultant on microscopy with a Nation Research Council grant of $25,000. But soon word got around the university of Naessens1 trouble with the medical authorities in France, and overnight the grant and Naessens' opportunity were gone.

It wasn't until 1971 that he could begin again as a medical researcher. A friend introduced him to David Stewart, scion of a tobacco fortune and head of the McDonald Stewart Foundation, which had funded unorthodox cancer research for many years.

After losing a dear friend to cancer, Stewart had vowed to pursue an avenue that might lead to a cure, and he was decreasingly confident of the conventional approaches the foundation supported. He agreed to finance Naessens' research personally, and established a laboratory for him on the McDonald Tobacco Company's premises in Montreal.

Naessens' run-ins with the French medical authorities, however, had forever branded him as a quack; his name was on the Quebec Medical Corporation's blacklist.

His new laboratory infuriated the orthodox oncologists under Stewart's wing, and they complained bitterly to the philanthropist. Stewart's response was to advise Naessens to move his research to some low-key spot and avoid getting embroiled in any more controversy.

Engaged by now to Francoise Bonin Sdicu, a divorced lab technician with four children, Naessens took over her family's summer cottage in Rock Forest, on the banks of the Magog river new Sherbrooke. He winterized and refurbished the place and built a lab in the basement.

Stewart's next concern was to get independent validation of the somatid theory and of the latest of Naessen's immune-system boosters, 714X; this was the nontoxic camphor-based medicinal designed to be injected by way of a lymphatic node in the groin, that was to figure in his trial in 1989.

Naessens had come to the conclusion - not essentially disputed by the orthodoxy - that cancer cells needed nitrogen to survive and "stole" this nitrogen from healthy cells.

Discovering that camphor had a natural, if inexplicable affinity for cancer cells, Naessens' biochemically linked a molecule of nitrogen to one of camphor, aiming to force-feed the rogue cells - which would leave the immune system free to rebuild itself and fight the cancer.

Excited by the potential of 714X, David Stewart approached McMaster University Medical Centre in Hamilton, offering to fund an investigative research project into Naessen's theory of the somatid cycle and the potential of 714X as an immune-system booster. The initial meeting at McMaster In March, 1972, went well.

The university was represented by Peter Dent, then chairman of the pediatrics department and consultant in immunology to the Ontario Cancer Foundation. But of all of those present to hear Naessens, the most impressed was a young assistant professor of pathology and surgery named Daniel Perey, who volunteered to head the proposed investigation, "The scope and the insight which Mr. Naessens has brought to this area of research potentially stand to benefit mankind and may be a source of pride for Canada."

Perey's first visit to Naessens lasted eleven days and was by all accounts a revelation to him; he saw through the somatoscope a new world to be explored.

The next time he brought Dent with him, assuming that his excitement would be shared. But Dent was clearly not happy to look through a microscope and see something that contradicted the definitions of disease he'd learned in medical school.

On returning to Hamilton, he wrote to the National Cancer Institute of Canada requesting its opinion of Naessens and his work. The institute sent him a page taken from a longer report it had published called Unproven Methods of Cancer Treatment. The page concentrated on an account of Naessens' trial in France and subsequent fine levied. This curt dismissal of Naessens' work confirmed Dent's unease.

But it was still Perey, not Dent who was conducting the investigation, and his enthusiasm for the somatid theory remained undiminished. Over the course of several visits to Rock Forest, Perey observed each of the forms in the somatid cycle proliferating and their apparent relation to cancer and other serious stresses on the body.

He recommended that Stewart's foundation purchase specialized photographic equipment enabling Naessens to capture these marvels on film - which was done. But the most telling sign of Perey's commitment to Naessens' work was a letter he wrote to support Naessens' application for landed-immigration status in September, 1972.

Emphasizing to the government the need for new and imaginative approaches to the search for a cancer cure, Perey extolled Naessens' contributions to the field, ending: "The scope and the insight which Mr. Naessens has brought to this area of research potentially stand to benefit mankind and may be a source of pride for Canada."

Apart from helping to secure landed status for Naessens, this letter - a solid endorsement signed by an orthodox medical researcher - augured well for the future. Or so one would think.

Just over two years later, Perey wrote another letter to Naessens, enclosing with it a copy of his final report to the Mcdonald Stewart Foundation. The report rejected the somatid theory and Naessens' notion of bolstering the immune system to fight cancer.

Even so, Perey tried to reassure Naessens that the report was not a condemnation of his work, rather, he wrote, "We have come to different conclusions and interpretations based on the scientific evidence which we have gathered, although in many instances we have observed identical or similar phenomena as you have." What happened to change Perey's mind?

Late in 1972, Perey had been assigned other duties that effectively ate up the time needed to run the Naessens study. The day-to-day running of the project was passed on to a husband-and-wife team of researchers who were not in the least interested in proving the overarching theories Naessens has sketched. They were interested only in one large form of the somatid cycle that had been described as bacterium by German researchers who had isolated it in the 1930's.

The couple wished to study claims that this particular form had an effect on rheumatism. So, although all future reports to the foundation on the Naessens project were still signed by Perey, their content was now a product of the new researchers, who did not accept Naessens explanation for what they observed in live blood through the somatoscope. They dismissed the stage of the somatid cycle as "artifacts" produced by mistakes during the process required to observe them.

Perey, caught between two camps, wrote to Stewart that "microbiological dogmas are so entrenched in the couple's minds that they do not allow themselves the luxury of challenging them." More than that, however, he could not give.

After the McMaster stonewall, Naessens grew skeptical about the chances of the medical establishment's ever confirming his views - though his hopes rose briefly again in 1974 after Dr. Raymond Brown, a consultant for New York's Memorial Sloan Kettering Cancer Center, visited Rock Forest.

Brown sent a memo to the centre's director and to staff about Naessens: "What I have seen is a microscope that reveals with spectacular clarity the motion and multiplicity of pleomorphic organisms in the blood which are intimately associated with disease states.

"The implications... are staggering... It is imperative that what its inventor, a dedicated biological scientist, is doing, and can do, be totally reviewed. I am convinced that he is an authentic genius and that his achievements cut across and illumine some of the most pertinent areas of medical science. If the review of his work is confirmatory, this man should be brought to New York and given unlimited support and facilities to continue his research."

Dr. Brown returned to Rock Forest with an oncologist and a microscopist from Sloan-Kettering; the three eventually drafted and signed a second and longer memorandum that reiterated the first.

These two memos generated much excitement among the hierarchy at the celebrated centre until someone noticed that Naessens' name appeared on the American Cancer Society blacklist. Immediately the memorandums were repudiated, the concerns of cancer bureaucrats outweighing the first-hand observations of expert scientists.

In August, 1980, Naessens supplied 714X to Dr. Gaetan Jasmin, a professor of pathology and medicine at the University of Montreal, who was willing to embark on the standard animal-control test, injecting 714X into cancerous and noncancerous rats.

He found that the compound had no effect on the rodents' tumors, and his results were reported in the Mcdonald Stewart Foundation literature in 1982.

But Jasmin had refused to follow Naessens' protocol for use of the drug. He had injected the medicinal into the tumors themselves rather than the lymphatic system, a procedure he has decided was impossible. Jasmin had treated 714X as if it were a standard anticancer drug that essentially poisons either the cancer or the patient.

Naessen's whole terrain approach was designed to treat the symptom via the cause - the diametrical opposite of orthodox oncological approaches.

And so Naessens' reputation continued to be vilified among the cancer researchers - which may have served only to recommend him to the desperate underground of cancer patients. Through the 1970's and 1980's more and more people flocked to his knowledge hoping for a personal miracle.

Through the 1970s and 1980s, more and more people flocked to Rock Forest, hoping for a personal miracle. And doctors began to come, eager to learn more about Naessen's new biology. Fully aware of the penalties for practicing medicine without a license, Naessens was not capable of turning away anyone who needed help. The suffering were taught to inject themselves with 714X, or referred to doctors who were willing.

All this action was not lost on Augustin Roy, the head of the Quebec Medical Corporation. In his eyes Naessens had been a marked man the moment he had arrived from France; David Stewart's patronage had angered Roy but had also caused him to proceed with caution. In 1984 Stewart died suddenly.

On December 13 of that Year, the police and officers of the Quebec Medical Corporation raided Naessens' house and laboratory, seizing vials of 714X and some 150 medical files that would bring Naessens to trial in the Sherbrooke courthouse in 1989. He seemed doomed to the hinterlands of science.

I first traveled to Rock Forest in January, 1992, taking with me a friend who would be termed a high risk for cancer: His mother and one brother have died from the disease; his father and another brother are currently undergoing treatment for it.

An unlikely spot for a revolution in science, from the outside Naessens' laboratory looked like any other summer cottage. At -18° C, however, it was not summer, and the snow crunched and squeaked as we walked towards the second of two cottages in the compound.

An informal seminar for two American MDs was being held that day, and we were invited to attend. Two guard puppies yelped, and tried to lick our faces, as Daniel Sdicu, one of Naessens' four stepchildren, opened the door.

Inside in a room bare but for a long table and chairs, Naessens stood to greet us. Tall and imposing - even his stepchildren refer to him as "Monsieur Naessens" -- he was formally polite. Introduced to the two doctors from Vermont, we sat quietly and listened.

One of the doctors, Bradford Weeks, interpreted Naessens' French for the other, a gaunt, worried-looking man. Part of the discussions in progress involved a new modified version of the somatoscope that Naessens calls an "ultramicroscopic condenser," which - attached to any optical microscope and for a modest $3,000 will enable a doctor or scientist to perform basic aspects of blood analysis according to the somatid theory. The rest covered what was to me by now familiar ground, with Naessens acting the strict but fair teacher.

Then we crunched fifty yards through the snow to the older, main cottage. Inside this neat and tiny house -- clearly Naessens' home --

we removed our boots, were given woolen slippers to wear, and were shown into a sitting room whose most prominent feature was an illuminated shrine to the Virgin Mary.

In one corner of this otherwise ordinary room a staircase led down. At the foot was a real if somewhat antique laboratory: Test tubes, retorts, specimen tubes, the lot. To one side, dominating everything, was the somatoscope. Looking like a cross between an ordinary large optical microscope and the inside of an old television set, the revolution in microscopy was definitely complicated.

A metal box labeled Helium-Neon Laser was attached to one side and a small video camera to the top; a web of wires ran to other contraptions below and behind it; there was a computer to the left, and some high-tech electronics connected to a monitor and Super VHS machine on the right.

Wandering down the long narrow room, with its panoramic views of the Magog ice scape, I came across a strange fleshy pink blob under clear viscous liquid in a sealed jar, like something left over from a David Cronenberg movie.

I asked the worried-looking Vermont doctor what it was. He peered closely at the slimy bolus and eventually replied, "I don't know, but whatever it is it's alive." Naessens cheerfully explained that the blob had started life as a bit of muscle tissue he'd taken from a living rat, injected with a concentration of pure rat somatids, sealed in a sterilized glass jar under vacuum, and then put on his lab windowsill back in 1978. "Ever since," he added, "the cells have continued to grow." "Great," the doctor laughed uneasily. "Grow your own hamburger."

What everyone was really here for, however, was to see his own blood under the unique microscope. First taking a sample from Dr. Weeks -- washing his hands, sterilizing the doctor's finger with alcohol, then taking the crimson pinprick onto a slide and covering it with a sliver of glass -- Naessens moved to his extraordinary device, flipping switches, positioning; the slide, peering through the eyepieces.

After focusing, he flipped another switch and the nearby monitor suddenly revealed what he was seeing. Tiny star-like dots pulsed and danced around brilliant circles that were, the biologist explained, red corpuscles. An awed silence followed, then gasps of amazement -- there was a singular beauty to this spectacle.

Carefully shifting the slide around -- the tiny pinprick of blood at 20,000 X like a hot tub full of stars - Naessens explained the various forms we saw in normal and healthy living blood, untreated, unstained.

Then it was the worried doctor's turn. There was the wait as the slide was prepared. But this time the blood looked distinctly different: The level of pulsing somatids seemed greatly reduced, and the later forms of the sixteen-stage cycle we're clearly present, some great twisted shapes, bars, and curious blobs with filaments.

"This is so strange," the doctor murmured, "seeing your own blood. I mean your own blood alive." Naessens scanned the sample more thoroughly than he had Dr. Week's. He asked if the doctor had been suffering from fatigue (he had) and the doctor in turn asked a few questions about AIDS that seemed to indicate the source of his worry.

Avoiding any explicit diagnosis, Naessens told him that there was definitely a stress on his immune system and that he should cut down his workload, rest more, and put himself on a strict diet - no red meat, no dairy products, lots of fresh fruit and vegetables. Then get his blood checked again in a month or so.

The man's mounting gloom was contagious; it also seemed a rather private moment to have strangers present, so my friend and I left, arranging to come back the next day. Neither of us could shake the image of that doctor faced with a picture of his mortality.

The next day it was my blood Naessens looked at first. With sweaty palms and a knotted heart, I waited until the video monitor was flipped on, seeing that universe of stars and red corpuscles like jostling balloons. Naessens moved the slide, pointing out forms, each one of which had me asking if that meant cancer. But no, all was as it should be. Beyond an apparent indication of iron deficiency Naessens saw nothing amiss.

Once I was able to relax, there was something inexpressibly thrilling about the play of the elements in living blood, my blood -- something fundamental.

But the mood was shattered. My friend's blood appeared next on the monitor. The red corpuscles seemed more frail and less defined. And stretching across the screen, coiled and serpent-like, was the last form in the sixteen-stage cycle - the "thallus," the discarded shell that has expelled new somatids. As Naessens moved the slide, indicating other forms from the complete cycle, my friend paced the lab in shock and fear.

Naessens continued to scan, pointing out forms, one of which -- a circular shape with waving snake-like protrusions that he termed the Medusa head -- seemed busy surrounding "intruders" or seemed at least very busy. "Ask your most eminent hematologists what that is," Naessens told me. "They cannot answer."

When my friend emerged from a prolonged and silent spell in the washroom, Naessens assured him that all this activity showed that his immune system was fighting, certainly, but in good shape. The somatid level was still relatively high, and the presence of the Medusa heads indicated an aggressive response to some form of stress.

My friend then told Naessens his family history, but the biologist still resisted any diagnosis, and advised him to follow the same regiment of diet and relaxation he'd recommended for the doctor the day before.

Augustin Roy had accused Naessens of furtive and covert work but Naessens was hardly secretive, his lab and files patently open to anyone who was interested. No-one was getting rich here either. When I asked if he's supplied 714X free to anyone willing to perform standard animal tests he immediately said yes, providing the tests were carried out according to his protocols, the compound injected intralymphatically and not into the tumors or the blood.

In Canada, because of his problems, Naessens was giving it away to any physician who asked for it through official channels. As of October, 1992, 210 M.D.s across the country were administering it to patients, admittedly on compassionate grounds, in most cases, and at their patients' request.

In retrospect, what impressed me most during this first exploratory visit was the devotion of Naessens' stepchildren. Only in Rock Forest did I learn that their mother, Francoise, had died of a rare fungal infection just four months earlier.

It was one of those horrible ironies that Naessens, who had helped so many people in endgame situations, had been unable to help his wife. Her children's faith in their late mother's strange and brilliant husband seemed absolute. That two of his stepchildren had degrees in biology said more for Naessens than any other fact of his life.

Shortly after we left, my friend's anxiety gave way to rage. How could I have subjected him to this? How could Naessens be so irresponsible as to put anyone through such an ordeal? Before we drove home, we went back to Naessens again, who went out of his way to reassure my friend that the apparent stress affecting his bodily system could easily be corrected at such an early stage. Hearing, once again, about the diet he should follow, my friend just groaned, "But what's left to eat?"

Never did a man follow a diet so religiously as did my friend over the next three months. And what I did, almost as religiously, was take the video tape of our blood and a description of Naessens' theories to anyone I thought might help me judge them.

Calling Tak Mak, head of cellular and molecular biology at the Ontario Cancer Institute, and one of this country's most eminent cancer researchers, I was surprised to find him unwilling even to hear an account of Naessens' work.

"it doesn't sound kosher," was all he said, adding that blood wasn't really his field anyway. He referred me to a leading hematologist at the OCI, Dr. Mark Minden, who reluctantly agreed to meet me and view the video tape shot through the somatoscope. Arriving early, I found Minden rummaging around his tiny cluttered office in jeans and sneakers. He claimed to have forgotten the appointment; he then left the room on the lookout, he said, for a VCR.

He came back half an hour later, without the equipment and patently hoping that I'd be gone. Instead I suggested that the nation's finest cancer-research hospital might have an audiovisual department. Muttering about grant applications that needed his urgent attention, he finally led me up many stairs and down many corridors to a cupboard possessing a monitor and a VCR into which I plugged my tape.

"What were the somatids?", I asked. "Platelets or proteins in Brownian motion", he replied, but I could see that something on the tape fascinated him. Did he ever study live blood? No — or very rarely -- was the answer. The electron microscopes and ordinary optical microscopes he used required fixed and stained blood.

To prevent his running out of the cupboard — he hopped from foot to foot like an athlete about to make the hundred -yard dash - I fast-forwarded to my friend's blood, asking him about the difference between the samples. Well, he said, this blood was obviously in an advanced state of clotting.

When I assured him that the sample had been taken under the same circumstances as my own, he pointed out that blood clots at different rates, though he'd have to look at it under the electron microscope to be sure of what he was seeing. What were the large coiled forms that Naessens identified as the final stage in the somatid cycle? Fibron, he said, a protein that forms when blood begins to clot. Why was there none of it in my blood sample, even after ten minutes of watching? He had no answer to that.

What Minden couldn't attribute to clotting he called "artifacts"-- a scientific way of saying "bits of stuff." The term in microscopy also implies structures that are accidentally created in the human handling of the sample on the slide. We looked at the Medusa head - the form Naessens had told me to show to a top hematologist.

He would have to stain and fix it to see if it had a nucleus, before he could comment; it was the only artifact that seemed to shake his certainty. I then showed him a diagram of Naessens' somatid cycle, which he dismissed outright. As I left Minden I thought, well, at least when pushed into a closet he was willing to look.

It took a while to find a doctor with an orthodox scientific background who was willing to stand up for Naessens. Dr. Dietmar Schildwaechter is an MD and medical Ph.D. who was a longtime faculty member of the University of Pennsylvania School of Medicine, the oldest medical school in the U.S.

One of his special fields was early cancer detection; he left the university to take over the Ratzenburg Klinik fur medizinische Rehabilitation, one of the world's most advanced cancer-rehabilitation centres, in his homeland, Germany. He now operates an office in the District of

Columbia consulting in preventive medicine and oncology while continuing to care for patients in Europe.

Schildwaechter came across Gaston Naessens in 1990 after discovering they were both treating the same "celebrity" patient, a "relative of George Bush". In 1986 the woman was diagnosed with "one of the most devastating cancers: an oat-cell carcinoma of the lung that had metastasized to the brain, the adrenal gland, and the tissue between the lungs," says

Schildwaechter. She and her husband had investigated the available treatments and discovered that for such a cancer there was no statistical survival after three years, though the rare individual did survive. Electing to go to the leading clinic in Bonn, she received chemotherapy, radiation, and various other primary treatments that brought the disease under control.

Then she was referred to Schildwaechter, who kept her on a maintenance program, employing frequent cancer and immune-system profile tests developed by Dr. Emile Schandl, a Hungarian-born research biochemist and geneticist who lives in Florida.

The monitoring-test results - immune parameters, complete blood count, differential count, blood chemistry, and so on - were computerized, giving, over the years, some of the most exact documentation of the results of the treatment of this illness that exist. "At the end of 1989," Schildwaechter says, "her blood sample arrived and its values had changed remarkably.

The immune-system values had improved drastically. We had always seen a slight activity from her cancer, which we'd kept in remission now it was down to zero. There were also two other markers that could not be done during this testing because, as our lab said, of something like chemical interference in her metabolism."

Schildwaechter called the couple to find out if something had been going on and found out that they had visited Naessens in Quebec, where the man had been taught how to give his wife injections of 714X. "They did not want to tell me because they thought I might not approve." They needn't have worried.

Schildwaechter finally met Naessens at a seminar held at Sherbrooke in 1991, and he unreservedly accepted Naessen's theory. At medical school in Europe he'd learned about Bechamp and others "basically excluded from medical schools over here. We were prepared for something like this," he says. "I knew there was something in the blood we'd not been able to diagnose, and I realized that Naessens had discovered and identified what others had only partially seen."

The resistance to Naessen's work from orthodox practitioners was only to be expected. Schildwaechter himself had been "a totally orthodox, tunnel-vision MD who didn't want to look at anything out of the mainstream" when he had been at the University of Pennsylvania. But then as he practiced he had begun to feel increasingly frustrated with the limits of his profession: "I had the most modern hospital, I could purchase the best equipment, yet I was still unable to monitor what I wanted."

In his spare time Schildwaechter traveled the world visiting medical centres and studying their techniques for monitoring blood, finding that none of them, from Britain to the Philippines, had the specificity and sensitivity that he required. "I could not in all conscience tell my patients that they were free of cancer after a monitoring test that was only sixty-five-per-cent accurate."

Then he met Schandl and, in a sense, defected from regular medicine: "Colleagues I had worked with for years were not even willing to discuss this stuff, even though Schandl was a leading biochemist and his test results were couched in all the proper forms." In Schildwaechter's view, his colleagues' excuse for dismissing Schandl's testing was that it was too complicated and impractical for ordinary labs to achieve.

The real reason, he believes, was that Schandl's tests could document the workings of alternative therapies that regular medicine had long dismissed and violently resisted. The future of medicine in Schildwaechter's eyes lies in prevention, and the essence of prevention is a greater understanding of the workings of the immune system and the development of methods to detect telltale signs of imbalance long before symptoms appear.

Combining, as he now can do, Schandl's tests with Naessen's somatoscopic monitoring, and something known as cell-milieu medicine - which determines the patient's exact needs for trace elements, amino acids, and vitamins.

Schildwaechter claims tremendous success with his German practice in detecting and correcting imbalances that would lead to degenerative diseases. (He hesitates to practice in the

U.S. for fear of Naessens-style prosecutions.) "Cancer," he announced with absolute conviction, "has become a truly preventable disease if we would only employ these blood tests.

"The number-one cancer today is breast cancer, so we tell women to have mammograms after forty. But regardless of how modern the equipment, there is still a high false-negative ratio and by the time the mammogram detects something, we've lost two years during which we could have prevented the cancer if the somatoscopic blood tests had been used."

Naessen's day is coming, insists Schildwaechter: "A number of oncologists are impressed with his work, even if they won't admit it at the moment." He sighs, and adds, "Szent-Gyorgyi, the discoverer of ascorbic acid and one of the great Nobel Laureates, remarked that whenever you pioneer something you first have to realize you may be called a quack. But the Establishment will check you out, and if they find your discovery useful it will be accepted through the 'back door' - certainly without giving credit to the-pioneer."

After three months' effort I did find two cautiously curious souls who were willing to look at the material through the back door and very much off the record. Even more off the record, they described Naessen's work as interesting, but hesitated about coming to Rock Forest with me to see the somatoscope in action.

Finally, I found a young microbiologist, Jacqueline Conant, then working as an associate scientist with the Robert Wood Johnson Pharmaceutical Research Institute in Toronto, who was intrigued (and professionally brave) enough to make the trip with me - and one very nervous friend heading for his second appointment with his own blood.

The moment Naessens had drawn the blood in question and turned to slide it into the jaws of the somatoscope, that friend was heading up the stairs, Naessens flipped on the monitor, revealing a vastly improved picture. He laughed and shouted, "C'est meilleur!" calling my friend back.

The full cycle of somatids was no longer evident, and the red corpuscles seemed more defined, more robust. The fast-clotting blood, as Dr. Minden had described it, had changed its nature in three months.

Next, Naessens showed us a video tape of blood from a patient with very advanced cancer. If normal blood had a sparkling beauty to it, this murky broth of filaments and tendrils had something deeply depressing about it. All the sixteen stages in the somatidian pleomorphic cycle were clearly visible, floating like wreckage in the blood. I couldn't see anything resembling red corpuscles and asked Naessens if this were so. He pointed them out - bubbles filled with grit, their edges jagged filaments.

Then Naessens played a tape of the same patient's blood after three months' treatment with 714X; after six months and a year. The progress was clear and dramatic. From what looked like Kitts's last cough, the final tape revealed that bright dancing universe I'd come to recognize as life and health. My friend was cheered, more at seeing what diabolically cancerous blood looked like than at this unknown patient's restoration to health.

Jacqueline Conant had looked at everything with obvious fascination, asking many questions in tolerable French, but it was only on the way back home that I was able to find out what had been going on in her mind.

"It was like entering the last century going down there," she said. "It reminded me of Banting and Best's lab at the U. of T. Then in the middle of it all, there's this feat of high-tech engineering through which he is able to make some truly remarkable observations." But what did she think he was seeing?

"It's never been possible to see these particular entities before - and I call them entities because they do appear to be living. What's their nature?" she asked. "They could possibly be fragments of genetic material, all right, but what exactly is their biochemical structure?"

One of the things Naessens had shown her was an electron-microscope photograph of a sectioned somatid taken at 140,000 X; it resembled something Norval Morrisseau could have painted. "I've never seen anything like it," she said, choosing her words with great care. "I certainly didn't recognize it to be of viral origin. It had definite structure, not structure as we normally know it, with a nucleus. But there was definite order to this particular structure."

Could it be, as Naessens maintained, a precursor to DNA?

After a long silence, Conant replied, "It is conceivable. It's the particular building blocks of DNA that one has never yet been able to visualize. In the electron microscope we've seen certain genetic fragments, chromosomes - the structures are fairly well elucidated."

A mighty pause. "I have trouble with that term precursor, but I suppose, yes, it is conceivable." Then, with passion: "There are so many tools around today that we would be able to elucidate a lot of Naessen's work, and yet the exciting thing for me is the extraordinary power of that particular microscope."

For microbiologists such as herself, she said, "it would certainly permit better patient management and therapeutic monitoring. There are really all kinds of exciting applications for such a device both diagnostically and academically."

She paused again, and frowned thoughtfully. "He was certainly able to show that many of the various examples of forms in the blood are quite disease-specific." Naessens had shown her still photographs of somatid" forms in the blood of AIDS, cancer, and multiple-sclerosis patients.

I told her Dr. Minden had described most of the forms as artifacts, and asked if the term did mean "bits of stuff." She laughed and said it did. But where did the stuff come from, I wondered, and why was there such a regular pattern in its forms? Could it all be the result of human handling of the samples?

She looked at me, gauging how far she wanted to go in her answer, and then, apparently, decided to jump: "There was very little manipulation between taking the blood, making the slide, and then viewing it. That's why there has to be something in it, and it certainly warrants further study. But it's so foreign to the accepted dogma, you know, that it's going to be a hard sell."

Perhaps Naessens will live long enough to see a front-door vindication of his life's work, in 1990, after receiving the positive results of non-toxicity tests, Health and Welfare Canada agreed that 714X could be supplied by Naessens to doctors whose patients were suffering from terminal cancer. Doctors have to apply to Ottawa, where authorities may try to talk them out of using it, but such requests now cannot be refused.

Naessen's frustration lies in not having approval for the medicinal's use in the early or precancerous stages of the disease, where he thinks it might be of the most use. But even with terminal patients he has begun receiving reports indicating that 714X helps relieve pain and restore energy during a patient's final days or weeks.

As far as his troubles with the Quebec medical authorities go, they've resulted in a temporary draw. Naessens and his lawyer, Conrad Chapdelaine, decided to fight back against the eighty-two counts that were laid after his first trial.

They countersued, issuing subpoenas to Augustin Roy, among others. The medical college replied with a plea-bargain offer, and in the end dropped seventy-two of the counts and reduced Naessen's fine to $5,000. Naessens and his lawyer regarded the outcome as a technical victory, and so far, there have been no more initiatives on the part of the authorities.

There is also growing interest in Naessen's approach to AIDS; he was invited to the controversial conference on alternative treatments held in Amsterdam last May - also attended by Luc Montagnier, the French scientist credited with discovery of HIV.

In Europe, the Philippines, New Zealand, and Australia, physicians are using 714X, and researchers, covertly and overtly, are investigating his work. Daily, results come in - favorable and unfavorable - the conclusion being that 714X does work most effectively when the immune system has not been totally wrecked by disease.

This has always been Naessen's contention. And as the new biology and the new medicine emerge, the textbooks will be rewritten, as they always have been, this time the emphasis shifting from cure to prevention.

An eminent Canadian oncologist (whom I will do the courtesy of not naming) has recently agreed, after visiting Rock Forest at my suggestion, to supervise certain tests to validate Naessens's somatid theory, an action that could jeopardize his career if publicized.

In the U.S., an independent study on 714X using human patients, sponsored by Charles Pixley, from Rochester, N.Y., has been underway since January of 1992.

In the Eastern Townships the man who may well be recognized one day as a Galileo or an Einstein continues the work, he has devoted half a century to, seemingly unconcerned by the fuss, the orthodox hostility. He works in silence and concentration in his laboratory, its windows on the Magog showing a landscape scarcely changed since the glaciers retreated.

Others have begun to praise him, but he himself might be content to live by a line from Paracelsus: "I pleased nobody except the people I cured."

This article originally appeared in **SATURDAY *night*, Canada's Magazine,** (circulation, 3,500,000), published in Toronto, Ontario, December 1992 issue.

Paul William Roberts, an author and freelance journalist from Toronto, received the Canadian "Journalist of the Year" award for this article.

AMERICAN ASSOCIATION OF NATUROPATHIC PHYSICIANS (A.A.N.P.) SYMPOSIUM

September 2, 1992.

The following is a transcription of Gaston Naessens' keynote address to the AANP Annual Conference at the Buttes Hotel in Tempe Arizona.

Gaston Naessens: (Translated from the French). Ladies and Gentlemen and dear friends. First of all, let me thank Christopher Bird for his eulogistic introduction, but equally he deserves thanks for the book he has written which permitted me to ventilate the somatid theory to the world.

Likewise, thanks to the AANP for their support and coverage of these new approaches. I am honored to be a part of this conference today. Now it is timely to review the results of the research.

Also, I propose a presentation which will be made by the Canadian team, first Andre Sdicu who is one of the administrators of The Center for Somatidian Orthobiology of the East (C.O.S.E.) who is in charge of the information and distribution of didactic and therapeutic material related to the somatidian theory.

I propose then for this morning that I shall explain to you the theory, the methodology, then the associated therapeutics of 714X. This afternoon we will see the clinical aspect, the influence of the somatidian theory on health and then a period of questions. I understand a little English, but I don't speak it. So, I pass the microphone to Mme. Levesque.

He then introduces Mme: Jacinthe Levesque, doctor/Df traditional Chinese Medicine, acupuncturist and director of the Center for Health specializing in alternative approaches for chronic and degenerative diseases.

Mme. Jacinthe Levesque (addressing the conference and translating for Gaston Naessens])

First I would like to say, you will hear things that Mr. Naessens has said and it might sometimes seem like the assertions are quite strong but you have to understand that what he is saying is based on forty years of research and since we're here to give you the good elements of all this we're not going to go into all the details or all the technical part of the microscope.

We want you to know that he, in 1949, as a microbiologist was looking at the blood and he was very curious because there were some particles, he was finding that were moving around and nobody seemed to know what they were.

So, from curiosity to creativity he has slowly been trying to create a tool which he calls the somatoscope, that would let him look at these particles. The somatoscope is basically an optic microscope that has a magnification power of 30,000X. So, what you will be seeing later in the video is part of what we can see in his somatoscope, but please understand that here today we are not using this device.

We are using an ordinary microscope with a special condenser to make sure that everybody will be able to see the somatids. Also, what we will see in the video is the cycle of the somatid that he has been able to identify in culture. Afterward we will see what happens when we look into the blood because when we look at a fresh blood sample, we don't necessarily see all sixteen stages.

I think it might be useful to review the principal characters of the somatid which you have seen in the cycle. First in a healthy state you have a micro cycle which can be seen and as soon as the blood inhibitors start to weaken or be in less concentration in the blood. Then the macrocycle starts to pick up and the complete cycle can be observed.

One of the major things that the experimentation with the chylomicron and the HDL can show you is that somatids really exist. That's one of the major arguments that the scientific community brings up.

People ask if the Taiuin method has been done. It has been done but since it takes another slide placed on top, it is not very conclusive. We could say that anything has been added so M Naessens would rather work with heat so that you can see the exact experimentation.

First: The Somatids major characteristic is that it is indestructible. It cannot be killed either by heat or by any chemical product. Secondly: The Somatid has to be present in any kind of cellular division. The somatid permits the growth hormone and that permits the cell to divide correctly.

He also has noted that somatids are electro-charged particles. The membrane has a negative charge, the nucleus has a positive charge and this can be verified by putting the positive pole of a magnet near the slides; all the somatids are attracted to the positive pull of the magnet.

Also, there is a repulsion movement which you can see when they come close to one another, indicating that they are electrically charged. M. Naessens thinks the somatid is the precursor of the ONA. He believes, it does not have all the same characteristics of the DNA, but it is a carrier of the genetic code.

Composition of the somatid: It is probably the link between energy and matter. Energy can take many forms. The somatid may be the link between the biological sciences and the physical sciences. We would like to explain the application of this theory.

In the beginning Mr. Naessens had a lot of opposition to his theory because there was only one tool, so he decided to put on the market a tool that would enable everyone with a dark field microscope to work with-this method.

Once he had identified the cycle, and after a lot of clinical observation and pathological experience with patients, he wanted to bring some kind of therapeutic action with a product. That's when the 714X was invented. It was a logical progression.

He wanted a product that had no side effects. He wanted a product to be put into the body that would be altogether natural. Moreover, he wanted a product that could be easily made under prime clinical conditions. The product contains camphor molecules, nitrogen molecules and organic salts. The camphor has a major role because it has a high power of attraction to the cancerous cell.

The 714X doesn't work to kill the cancerous cell. It works to attract certain activities around the cancerous cells so the immune system can recognize it, for people in traditional Chinese medicine we know that the camphor has a high power on the chên. He then charged this cancer molecule with nitrogen because he had observed that cancer cells are very greedy for nitrogen and they will steal nitrogen from the healthy cells.

Now that the cancer cell is highly attracted to the 714X, the third ingredient, the salts, serve to liquefy the lymph. He has noted that all persons with degenerative diseases have a gelatinized, or clogged lymph.

So being able to function normally, the lymphatic system can do its job and carry away the toxins out of the body. The 714X is injected into the lymphatic system directly.

The cancer cell in order to steal nitrogen from the healthy cell secretes what Mr. Naessens calls a co-cancerogenic K factor which paralyzes and blocks or makes it invisible to the immune system. When the cancer cells have all the nitrogen they need, they cease to secrete this factor.

After ten or fifteen days of injections we start to see the immune system starting to respond and begin doing its job. Thus, the camphor compound serves as a diversionary tactic to distract the cancer cells until the immune system is strong enough to begin carrying away the cancerous toxins. This is a simplified explanation of the activity of 714X.

QUESTIONS AND ANSWERS

Question 1; Aren't you making the cancer cells grow by giving them nitrogen?

Answer: Since you are giving all the nitrogen wanted to the cancerous cells, they are not secreting the K factor that blocks the immune system. So, while you are feeding them, they are not doing anything detrimental to the body, they are just feeding so you are giving a good chance to the immune system to pick up so the liquefied lymph can carry off the toxins.

Question 2: While the cancer cell is eating nitrogen is it in a-latent state or does it continue to reproduce?

Answer: It can continue to reproduce for a certain while until the immune system can pick up. It takes a critical mass of cancer cell to make it secrete the [co-cancerogenic] K factor that paralyzes the immune system, so the whole idea is to decrease this critical mass. As long as it is not secreting the K factor to gain nitrogen, the immune system is repairing itself and will eventually take over.

Question 3: Are there other factors that will paralyze the immune system besides the K co- factor.

Answer: There is no other factor that will paralyze the immune system. The only thing that can change is the inhibitors. Inhibitors are sensitive to the way we eat, the way we live, etc. So, the inhibitors in the blood being in less quantity will allow the macrocycle to begin and when the macrocycle starts it is the K co factor that will block the immune system.

Question 4: Is the somatid the smallest living organism?

Answer: Not only is it the smallest living unit, but I believe it is the link between cosmic energy and first manifestation of matter. Somatids are in liquid form inside the red blood cell. When it is healthy, it is as though the red blood cell will secrete that liquid form in the plasma and the somatid will just take form, and materialize in the plasma.

Otherwise in certain types of disease, the somatid will materialize inside the red blood cell; so that's another indication that something is wrong.

The micro cycle of the somatid which is the normal three stage cycle, liberates a growth hormone that is necessary for cell division.

Question 5: What constitutes the somatid? Is it a blood inhibitor?

Answer: The somatid is a particle with a cycle that is influenced by blood inhibitors. We can have a high concentration of somatids and a low amount of blood inhibitors.

Question 6: Does the 714X replace the blood inhibitors?

Answer: The 714X brings the macrocycle back to the microcycle and to do this you need a certain amount of blood inhibitors which are activated by an increasingly healthy immune system.

Question 7: Do the growth hormones cause the somatid to go from the microcycle to the macrocycle?

Answer: The blood inhibitors are usually a barrier and they stop the growth hormones from moving [the somatid] past the first three cycles [into the macrocycle].

If there are no blood inhibitors then the cycle starts to pick up and can move very fast.

The whole cycle can be completed in 92 hours.

Question 8: Does the somatid secrete the growth hormone?

Answer: It is not the somatid that secretes (he growth hormone. It is the transformation of the somatid that liberates the growth hormone, but it is not a secretion of the somatid.

The somatid originates in a liquid form inside the red blood cell. Each transformation of the somatid generates a new secretion of growth hormones.

Question 9: What are the blood inhibitors?

Answer: Blood inhibitors could be vitamins, organic salt, that is anything in the chemistry of the blood that is going to stop this process [of growth from the microcycle to the macrocycle]. They can be influenced by the way you eat, the way you live, your emotions. This is the holistic approach. This we will see in the other video, what we have to do to keep the blood inhibitors in good shape.

Question 10: What are the organic salts that are used in the 714X compound?

Answer: Mostly ammonium chloride. When there is no ammonium chloride the albumen of the lymph starts to be clogged up.

Question 11: Potassium?

Answer: No.

Question 12: What is the correlation of concentration of somatids in the blood before and after 714X?

Answer: The concentration of somatids in the blood cell is an indicator of health of the natural mechanism of defense. The somatid is a particle on its own. It is something in the blood system that can work to either paralyze or help your immune system.

Question 13: What amount of time does it take to go from healthy microcycle to unhealthy macrocycle?

Answer: The length varies, it depends on blood inhibitors which are influenced by the way you eat, the way you live, stress, emotions, your own chemistry. It can be a matter of weeks, very short.

You have to understand what you can see in the blood regarding the cycles of the somatid. It can take a year for a body to develop a cancer. We can see the cycle of the somatid and you would be asymptomatic at that time. You can go for a checkup and they would never see anything wrong in your blood. This is why the method is good for preventive assessment.

The cycle can be seen 18 to 24 months before symptoms appear. Seeing in the microscope the stages of the cycle is not enough to confirm that the sickness is there. It is a biological indicator which must be considered with other factors.

[The macrocycle] is not a cause of the disease, but an indicator. At this stage you may not be sick. You might be tired, with a loss of vitality, confused and having non-specific symptoms. This is a sign that the critical mass of disorganized cells is increasing to the point where they will secrete the co K factor and affect the activity of the lymph.

Question 14: How does the 714X apply to other diseases like MS?

Answer: The same process goes on in any degenerative sickness indicated by stage four of the cycle.

Question 15: What is the connection between the macrocycle and the pathology that we normally see, in other words cancer or multiple sclerosis. Does the macrocycle cause the disease?

Answer: It is the indicator not the cause of something going wrong in the body.

Question 16: Is there a quantifiable correlation between the macrocycle and the pathology of disease in clinical documentation of cases treated?

Answer: In 1964 there were already 10,000 cases of different types of cancer treated, in a double-blind study in France. When you are looking at the blood of a patient with cancer you can find all these particles, same for multiple sclerosis, AIDS, or any type of degenerative disease.

A certain part of that cycle you will see in cancer patients, you will not for multiple sclerosis. So, we had to figure out what indication in that cycle will show us if the patient is going to develop MS or Epstein Barr. If you have a degenerative sickness you will see more elements of the terminal stage of the cycle, you will see phase 15 and 16, and a lot of them.

Question 17: Of all the many pleomorphic theories which have a therapeutic tool that is linked to it, do they all work in the same way?

Answer: I don't know all the other products specifically, but the 714X is the only product that liquefies the lymphatic system and permits the toxins to be carried away from the system and prevent metastatic activity of the cancerous cell.

Question 18: Does the camphor attract any other kind of cells?

Answer: Camphor attracts all cells preparing for degenerative disease, whether it be cancer, lupus, Epstein Barr or MS.

Question 19: What is your evidence that cancer cells like nitrogen and that in degenerative disease the lymphatic system is all clogged up?

Answer: That research has been universally done and is widely known in the field of biology, a principle called the nitrogen trap. M. Naessens has seen it, but he is not the only one to do so. The assertion about the lymph is possible because he did a lot of tests with lymphography trying to insert dye into the body of a person with degenerative disease, but he couldn't do it at all before treatment. After taking the 714X, within a minute this procedure could be done effectively. In clinical treatment you can see this with a patient. After having an injection, there is a heat flush after not even ten minutes as the lymph liquefies and begins to flow.

This came up in Los Angeles. People said we know that you can liquefy the lymph, either by massage or by electro-therapy and Mr. Naessens said yes this is true, we know this. We are not trying to push 714X. You can liquefy the lymph in other ways but you provide no long-term solution for the immune system and you run the risk of forcing toxins into the blood or into the lymphatic system and you are toxifying the system even more.

All he is saying is it's an effective way to liquefy the lymph naturally where the toxins are released naturally and the body feels it naturally and it is not forcing toxins into the system any faster than the body can handle it.

The 714X has had good results on the psychology of the person. We see that people open up and that emotions are more easily expressed. Some will see the physical aspects-- increased vitality, and some will see more openness in their emotions, but the liquefication of the lymph is the basic action.

The clinical doses are very progressive. We start with .1 and .2 cc. and increase systematically to .5 cc so that the toxins will be eliminated in a way that will not overtax the kidneys and other organs of elimination.

Question 20: For vitamin B12 and Vitamin E what doses are possible? How about megadoses?

Answer: In Mr. Naessens opinion megadoses are not recommended and in the case of B12 and E they should not be taken. B12 because it activates cell division and E provides a shield of protection around the cancer cell so that the immune system cannot attack it.

READING THE BLOOD

Question 21: How soon do you have to look at the fresh blood slide after it is drawn?

Answer: Immediately. Within ten minutes maximum.

Question 22: In dark field microscopy what can be seen that can't be seen in others?

Answer: You can see a different morphology of the cell like the polynuclear in the case of AIDS is completely different. You will have abnormalities in platelet where you see the bubble formation.

Also, in lymphocytes, the membrane changes and the cytoplasm are completely different. So, there is a difference. You can see in certain types of disease, usually in cancer, the red blood cell is parasitized. Sometimes you will see the membrane change to a crenated form. You have to be careful because sometimes dehydration can do the same thing.

Question 23: What is the clinical significance of the bubble in the platelet?

Answer: When there is a viral infection you can be sure this type of abnormality will start, from herpes to AIDS. When you find that in very large quantities, you can start looking for AIDS.

Question 24: Does it make a difference if you take a blood test after eating?

Answer: Yes, if you look at the somatids the number will seem to be increased. But mainly the lipoprotein and chylomicron will be fixed on the slide after twenty to twenty-five minutes, so you will see a difference after twenty to twenty-five minutes.

Question 25: What exactly can you eat within the diet guidelines?

Answer: Anything besides having things cooked in a lot of butter, or deep fried or anything that has fatty acids. The nutritional guidelines in the video are very general. For those with a good nutritional diet, they can continue same. The better the diet is the more quickly the immune system can pick up.

Question 26: Is there any form of administration of 714X other than injection? How are the doses figured?

Answer: Three major forms, peri-nodular injection, the best, the nebulizer and there are the oral drops. The same quantity is always given to the patient. Only with a child you must reduce the dosage. The maximum dosage with an adult is .5 cc a day and .3 cc for the child.

You can use a nebulizer, if a patient has a brain tumor, at the same time as the injection, but the injection is the best way to get the most out of the 714X. In the case where the right inguinal lymph node is removed, which happens frequently, you can use the left side. However, you will have a lesser result, or it will take more time. The lungs and the bronchus are filled with lymph nodes, that's why the use of the nebulizer can be effective.

Now concerning the oral drops that only goes to the blood stream, not the lymph nodes, so you will not have the same action. You can use oral drops for herpes and we have seen that in a short period of time the herpes will go away. For people with a bad cold or flu it is a good antiviral, used sublingually.

714X A HIGHLY PROMSING NON-TOXIC TREATMENT FOR CANCER AND OTHER IMMINE DEFICIENCIES

by Gaston Naessens, Biologist

When one views cancer as a cellular disease, isolated from general biological disorders and developing along proper norms which are local and independent of any possible carcinogen whose persistence is no longer indispensable to the autonomous progression of the tumoral process, the therapy is centered on the "tumoral mass" whose destruction and radical removal becomes the only imperative means of recovery.

Until now, among the means at our disposal for combating this disease, the surgical solution has figured most prominently. This solution, which best addresses the notion of "tumors as a local disorder," consists of the radical removal of the autonomous mass from the cellular agglomeration, which appears as an immediately palliative solution.

Next came the radiation solution. This therapy applied to tumors, which proposes the destruction of the tumoral mass by deep disintegration of the cancerous cells and for which the question of dosage and irradiated surface is an important consideration, would not be efficient other than to the extent in which the radiation would reach the neoplastic cells, not with the intent of immediate and blind disintegration but rather to force a reversal of the pathological synthesis which is the source of their malignancy.

Finally came the chemotherapeutic solution. The therapeutic solution based on the use of chemicals toxic to such cells, which is to say by karyoclasic poisons which stop the mitoses by plasmatic division and chromatic alteration, leads to duplications of the number of chromosomes and abnormal mitoses.

The karyoclasic action of this therapy appears, with regard to neoplastic mitoses, as an essentially negative mode of stopping, blockage, and chromial disintegration and furthermore presents a danger-without speaking of general toxicity—to the mitoses of normal cells and among others, to that of the germinal series.

NATURAL IMMUNITY

For some time already, a new orientation had been taken in the work of researchers studying cancer. As a matter of fact, the possibilities of natural immunity, as much zoological as physiological or individual in the cancer grafts, whose essentially anti-tissular nature remains obscure, have shown that cancer should no longer be considered a cellular disease isolated from general biological disorders.

To the contrary, the evolution of this disease is linked to conditions of the organism, and the aptitude to cancerization points back to the organism "alone."

To grow, the tumor needs the organism and without the latter cancerization cannot take place. Given the interaction which exists between the organ and the tumor, in particular its vascularization and the composition of the blood which irrigates it as well as the state of nervous influx pertaining to it, all modification of these different factors can thus have an action on the very life of the cancer.

The process which at certain times permits the host carrier of tumor to stabilize it, should be analogous to that which permits an individual to harbor in his throat diphtheria bacillus without being stricken by this disease.

It is possible that similar phenomena occur with regard to malignant cells. This is reasoning by analogy. If one considers the numerous possible causes of cancer which surround us, is it not possible that there exists in certain individuals, a resistance to the development of cancer?

GRAFTS STUDIES

A number of studies have been undertaken with the purpose of clarifying this problem. The first attempts were undertaken with patients stricken with advanced cancer, who had volunteered to undergo these experiments. Some tumor fragments, removed from other persons and cultivated for a long time in an artificial medium were implanted under the skin of their fore-arms. The grafts were accepted and progressively grew in volume.

This result was in contradiction with the usual biological rule which requires that a tissue removed from an animal does not develop itself if it is grafted-on another animal, unless the latter is a true twin of the first. The explanation of this statement, which appears to be paradoxical, requires that, with patients stricken with advanced cancer, the natural defense which opposes the acceptance of grafts had disappeared.

One could inquire further if all the usual defenses of these fatigued patients had thus given up. The experiment showed that the normal defense mechanism that yielded to the cancer, remained intact in all other respects. It is thus that a graft of normal tissue was rapidly eliminated.

The two possible explanations were that, either the cancerous tissue had a particular ability of growth contrary to the usual laws which rule grafts, or the patient had lost, especially with regard to cancerous cells, the possibilities of normal defense.

The question then was would cancer cells transplanted to a normal individual be capable of growing? A systematic study of this question had been undertaken by the cancer research center in New York, which called on volunteers from an American prison. From more than one hundred volunteers, fifty men were chosen. These men received an implant of a human cancer culture, the same type as that which had been utilized within the patients stricken with cancer.

With the fifty volunteers, there had been one important defensive local inflammatory reaction and the graft disappeared completely in four weeks. This experiment demonstrated that the human body possesses some type of resistance to the growth of cancers transplanted from another man.

This resistance does not exist with patients stricken by advanced cancer. These experiments lead one to attempt to stimulate the natural defense of an organism against cancer. This is why several researches were undertaken in the area of immunology.

It is a question of knowing if the elements which constitute the malignant tumor, essentially the chemical elements which form the cell or the nucleus, are capable of playing the role of antigen. This is to say, to provoke in the organism which contains them, the formation of antagonistic substances called antibodies, whose role it is to oppose the development of the former, or antigen.

If such a property can be disclosed in malignant tumors, it would indicate the possibility of promoting the formation of such antibodies for fighting against the development of cancer. The problem is not so simple though, because the normal tissues from which cancer results, are grafted on another subject. It is necessary to suppress the antibodies thereby formed in order to verify if other antibodies exist whose formation would be due to the presence of malignant tissue.

It would be necessary to admit that, not the tumor but perhaps one or several elements of the cell play the role of forcing the body in its development in the organism. It is possible to consider that in certain circumstances, there exists a certain degree of antigenic properties, and that it may then be possible to promote the development and encourage the formation of corresponding antibodies.

This phenomenon would then be able to explain why certain carrier subjects of cancer, although having diffused the cells from the primary tumor in the organism, do not lead to the development of other metastases. The cells stopped at other points could have provoked there the formation of antibodies which were opposed to their development or which could have destroyed them.

One can equally envision a lowering of immunity which had stabilized the swarming cells, thus allowing for the development of metastases years after the destruction of the initial tumor.

TUMOR CELLS

The problem of cancer viewed from this angle makes it necessary to study the life of the malignant cell in order to discover which antigenic agents would be capable of producing such antibodies as are capable of destroying cancerous cells.

Despite very particular aspects of the malignant cell, it is surprising to note that one may again ask how it can differ from a normal cell. Research seeking to put into evidence a new element not found in normal cells found no conclusive result.

On the contrary, it would seem that there are qualitative differences in the choice made by the cell between the primary materials which supply it in particular in the chemical phenomena and the fermentations leading to the formation of nucleic acids - the role of which is essential in the life of the cell.

Tumor cells utilize more glucose than normal cells, but no quantitative differences have been found between normal tissue and tumoral tissue. This strongly indicates an increase in the formation of lactic acid. Tumor cells utilize the energy produced by the destruction of carbohydrates for the synthesis of cellular proteins at a greater level than normal cells.

The cells return to a simpler form. The phenomena associated with fermentation (linked to ferments called enzymes), basic to proper life, simplify the cell, which then loses more or less those functions which individualize it and make it pertain to a specialized organ.

Before the cell has utilized all its capacity for synthesis, it divides, thus prematurely interrupting the cycle of its activities and aggravating the disorder at each division. In response, it recovers former properties remembered from its origin - most important of which is the aptitude to multiply more rapidly, with consequences which are one of the manifestations of its malignancy.

This abnormal growth in number is due to a liberation of the control system which normally maintains tissue harmony. The cells then become dangerous parasites or anarchists in the midst of the cellular community. The malignant cells appear "privileged and antisocial."

They first monopolize materials, and in particular, amino acids indispensable to the life of all cells, whether normal or malignant. What is especially striking is the intensity of these physical or chemical phenomena in comparison to ordinary chemical phenomena in normal conditions. The surrounding conditions, temperature, Ph and molecular pressure, have a capital importance on the phenomena of cellular life.

PHYSICAL STATE OF HUMORS

Of all the problems the most important is, without doubt, the disorders of the humoral system engendered by these phenomena and the consequences which come from the behavior of individuals in a normal or pathological state.

Hippocrates, and well before his time, "the Hebrews and the Egyptians, already attributed the major part of morbid incidents to troubled humors.

By "humors" we mean the extra-cellular liquids of the organism. They form the fluid part of the circulating blood: the plasma, in which the sanguine elements appear, such as the suspended white and red blood cells, and also all the interstitial liquids either lacunal or others, which bathe, impregnate or encircle the tissue and organs.

Not having a precise means of investigation, the ancients completely ignored how and why humors can be innovative. Later, when the constitution of these humors became known, medicine sought to discover which of the substances which compose these humors were responsible for the incidence of pathology.

Having identified that all experimentally provoked variations, in terms of diverse humorous constitutional elements, had been powerless to reproduce the symptoms of acute or chronic diseases, they came to this conclusion diametrically opposed to that of Hippocrates: "that the humoral state plays no role in the genesis of illness." Medicine then became "solidest": Only lesions were considered important; the state of humors was left aside.

On a modern basis, we will endeavor to recognize the triumph of humoral medicine in discovering the real reason for the innovative behavior of humors, which resides, not in their chemical constitution, but in the physical state of certain elements, when the latter ones change to the state of a solid.

We are drawn to examine the behavior of observable elements in all biological liquids, in particular our attention has been retained by extremely tenuous particles, whose presence has already been signaled by numerous authors in the end of the previous century.

For quite some time already, the microscope has been an indispensable instrument for precise measurement in research laboratories and the industry. The classical microscope normally permits enlargement on the order of 1800X with a resolution of 0.1 microns.

The electron microscope permits enlargement on the order of 400,000X with a resolution of 30 to 50 angstroms. But use of the latter necessitates manipulations which alter the physical aspect of objects being observed.

We have thus perfected an instrument of microscopic observation which we have called Somatoscope. The primary quality of this apparatus is that it permits the observation of live elements and can follow the polymorphism to enlargements attaining 30,000X with a resolution on the order of 150 angstroms.

Using this instrument, we have observed in all biological liquids and particularly in the blood, an elementary particle endowed with a movement of electronegative repulsion, possessing a polymorphic nature. We have called it "somatid." This extremely tenuous particle whose dimension varies from a few angstroms to 0.1 microns, can be isolated and put in a culture. We could then observe the polymorphic cycle shown in Figure 1. (ed., see p.)

We were surprised to discover in this cycle such elements which we had regularly seen in the blood of healthy persons but equally in the blood of carriers of diverse diseases. We made certain correlations.

In the blood of healthy persons, we observe somatids, spores and double spores. In the course of this micro-cycle we can detect the production of a "trephone." this is a proliferative hormone indispensable to cellular division. Without it, life does not exist. I healthy individuals, the evolution of this cycle is stopped at the level of the double spore because of the presence of trephone inhibitors in the blood, these are either mineral substances like copper, mercury and lead, or organic substances such as cyan-hydric acid, etc. In the course of this micro-cycle, the quantity of trephones necessary for cellular multiplication is thus elaborated.

If, because of stress or some biological disturbances, the inhibitors in the blood diminish in concentration, the somatid cycle continues its natural evolution and one sees the appearance of diverse forms of bacteria. These have also been termed by German scientists during the 1930's, as syphonospora polymorpha.

Next come the myco-bacterial forms, and then the yeast-like forms. These forms with a dimension of 4 to 5 microns evolved rapidly into ascospores, then by maturation become asci.

At this stage of evolution, the ascus, after staining on a blood smear, appears as a small lymphocyte and cannot be differentiated by conventional means.

Next come the filamentous forms. One can observe from an ascus, the formation of a thallus in which evolves a cytoplasm of increasing importance. The cytoplasm is formed from the ascus and a conjuncture is observable between them. It is by this conjuncture and by peristalsis that the cytoplasm forms in the thallus.

This apparent mycelial form responds to none of the criteria of fungal elements. In fact, it is in no way affected by massive doses of Amphotericin B, Fungizone or other antifungal agents.

When this pseudo-mycelial element has attained its full maturity with an extremely active cytoplasm, we then witness the bursting of this thallus and the liberation into the surroundings of an enormous quantity of new particles capable of re-initiating a complete cycle.

The empty thallus has a fibrous aspect. Furthermore, it is often seen on blood smears but it is considered as an artifact of the staining procedure.

From the preceding observations, we have been able to draw the following conclusions:

1. Cellular division requires the presence of the SOMATID (which is in both the animal and plant domain).

2. Trephones are elaborated by the SOMATID.

3. The SOMATID is capable of polymorphism. This polymorphism is controlled by inhibitors found in the blood.

4. A deficiency of sanguine inhibitors permits the elaboration of a large quantity of trephones, which in turn lead to disorders in cellular metabolism.

5. All degenerative diseases are a consequence of these disorders.

In light of the above observations, the notion of «cancer, a general disease, which is localized» takes on its meaning when one examines the evolution process of this affection. This process can be divided in two parts:

First part: Cancerization or initiation.

When, for whatever reason, the sanguine inhibitors and the polymorphism of the somatid is no longer stopped at the double spore state, an exaggerated formation of trephones in the organism leads the cell to return to a simpler form.

The phenomena of fermentation (linked to ferments called enzymes), basic to proper life, simplify the cell. It then loses more or less those functions which give it its individuality and make it pertain to a specialized organ.

The cell is divided even before it has utilized all its capacity for synthesis, thus prematurely interrupting the cycle of its activities and aggravating its disorder at each division.

In response it recovers old properties remembered from its origin - the most important of which is the ability to multiply rapidly, with consequences which are one of the manifestations of its malignancy. This abnormal growth in number is due to a liberation of the control system which normally maintains cellular harmony.

At this stage, the cancerization is effective.

It can be called initiation or precancerous. We now have an accelerated and anarchic multiplication of one or several cells which provokes, by an agglomeration of their descendants, the occurrence of a new «entity» opposing the organism which had given birth to it.

The immune system enters into action and fights actively to eliminate this entity. In this fashion, we develop a small cancer daily, but our immune system rids us of it.

Second part: Co-cancerization or promotion.

If the immune system is somewhat deficient and the new entity has been able to reach a certain proportion, then it attains a «critical mass» of cells in anarchic proliferation.

This entity which has been able to escape from the immune system, needs an enormous quantity of nitrogen for subsistence (the cells of this entity are moreover named Nitrogen Traps).

It then emits a substance which allows it to withdraw nitrogen derivatives from the organism and which at the same time, paralyses the immune system. We have called this substance Co-cancerogenic K Factor (C.K.F.).

The paralyzing action of C.K.F. against the immune system appears only when the critical mass of cells in anarchic proliferation is reached. From this moment, the organism finds itself without defense against this new entity which can develop at will and progressively invade its host.

We can conclude from this analysis that:

1. The cancerization or initiation phase is linked to the reduction of sanguine inhibitors and a weakness of the immune system.

2. The co-cancerization or promotion phase is the direct consequence of paralyzed immune system provoked by a substance call C.K.F. This substance is elaborated by anarchic cells in order to withdraw, from the organism, nitrogen derivatives necessary for proliferation.

The understating of this process makes it possible to propose a therapy leading to the suppression of C.K.F. As a matter of fact, if the latter is neutralized, the immune system can regain its initial activity and consider each anarchic cell composing the tumors as a foreign body to be rejected.

After having carried out numerous experiments on camphor and its derivative, we have discovered that this product is endowed with remarkable pharmaceutical properties since it impedes the formation of the C.K.F. substance, which puts leukocytes and other phagocytic elements of the organism in a state of negative chemotaxis, that is to say in a state of paralysis during diverse degenerative diseases.

Camphor is neither an antimitotic nor an antimetabolite. Its property of inhibiting the

C.K.F. resides in the fact that it carries to the tumors cells all the nitrogen which it needs, suppressing by the same action the secretion which would paralyze the immune system.

We have therefore proposed for experimentation a camphor derivative, TRIMETHYL BICYCLONITR AMINO HEPTANE-CL going by the brand name 714X.

***

"It's not the critic who counts. Not the man who points out where the strong man stumbled or where the doer of great deed could have done them better. The credit belongs to the man who is actually in the arena. Whose face is marred by dust and sweat and blood. Who strives valiantly, who errs and comes up short again and again. And, who, while daring greatly, spends himself in a worthy cause so that his place may never be among those cold and timid souls who have known neither victory nor defeat"

Theodore Roosevelt

SOMATIDIAN ORTHOBIOLOGY

Theory, Technique and Project protocol

This research project constitutes a format for the practical application of knowledge. Those participating in this project are patrons (from pater, -father), who actively support rather than patients (from pascho-suffer, endure), who passively suffer.

The Sponsors of this Project, named below, share the desire to provide an independent, international forum for the voice of reason and genuine scientific inquiry, research and synthesis.

Tracking and record keeping of the investigation.

All patrons will be offered the opportunity to take a series of blood tests based on HCG, PHI, GGTP, CEA and DHEA-S values to establish a "baseline" profile at the beginning and track progress during the treatment period.

The testing process will provide the patron, doctor and the investigators with information on the progression or regression of the patron's condition as well as provide appropriate records for the purposes of the investigation.

In some cases when applicable or possible there may be the use of a microscope and/or potential filming of blood samples and making of video copies of each patron's blood samples before, during and after treatment.

General Purpose and Guidelines of this Research Protocol

1) To make absolutely sure that the patrons participating in the investigation have adequate and complete information regarding the investigation and its potential risks, allowing them to make an informed decision prior to granting their written consent.

2) To assure that any drug or medical device and its protocol has acceptable standards which will allow it to be used in Hospitals and that the risks of the drug or medical device are exceeded by the potential benefits.

3) To determine the efficacy of 714X in treatment of HIV, AIDS and other immunological and degenerative diseases and gain a marketing permit.

The following conditions are included in the project protocol:

1) There will be use of a substance banned by the United States F.D.A., namely TRIMETHYLBICYCLONITRAMINOHEPTANE-CL, 714X. The 1994 Canadian Investigational and Emergency Drug List includes 714X for Anti-Cancer and Immune Related Disease Therapy.

2) (Drug Information Center, Ontario College of Pharmacists, Toronto, Canada)

3) There will be a direct cost to the participant for the substance and for the physician's services. Patrons will not receive any compensation for participation in this investigation.

4) The subjects will be enrolled in the project/protocol on a purely voluntary basis and only after they have read, signed and submitted the petition and consent application and their pertinent case history and obtained the assistance of an informed medical professional.

5) Human patrons will be subjects. There may be non-patron volunteers. There may be questionnaires. There will be no pregnant patrons, although there has been experience in treating a pregnant mother for cancer and the child was born with no complications. There will be subjects of all ages. There may be mentally disabled patrons.

6) Proteolytic enzymes may be used as well as other non-prescription, nutritional substances.

7) There may be approved drugs for new uses; however, none are specifically planned for this study. There may be devices, namely a syringe holder device to facilitate the injection process. The patrons may be advised or requested to use an ultrasonic nebulizer.

8) There will be no use of surgical, pathology tissue except possibly to track necrosis or tissue remission, etc.

9) To date, there are no known adverse side effects from the use of the 714X. Risks include the possibility that only partial or no benefit whatsoever is derived. Benefits are the possibility of improvement or complete and permanent remission of the existing condition.

10) Potential side effects or reactions that could arise from usage by intra or para-nodular injection is itching, a non-life threatening, burning sensation or post injection throbbing at the site of the injection and sometimes a feeling of exhilaration, or fatigue during the periods of the injections.

11) Should there be at any time an adverse reaction arising from the use of the medicine, your participation should be terminated or at least stopped until medical consultation.

12) Confidentiality will be maintained by customary means (anonymity of the subjects, etc.). However, the patrons will sign a consent form which will allow the pertinent data from each case to be sent to the Sponsors on a regular basis for use by the Board, always maintaining the anonymity of the patron.

13) (12 Consultation and exchange of patron consent forms will ensure that information is available to the patient's primary physician if he is other than the investigator, as per the informed and written consent of the patron.

14) There will be no placebos.

Camphor is a primary active component of the 714X compound. Medical References to Camphor

<u>ORIENTAL MATERIA MEDICA</u>, 1936, 1st Edition, pages 772

Compendium of Empirical Medical References by Hong Yen Hsu. Specific references reveal a five-thousand-year history of usage up to and including 1.5 grams per dose for oral use.

<u>BOERICKE and RUNYON</u>, 9th Edition, 1927, pages 158-160

References to camphor appear in Boericke and Runyon since the late 18th Century and refer to the original teachings of S. Hahnemann, physician and founder of Homeopathy, published in The Organon. Hahnemann recommended its use in the treatment of "Scabies, Cholera, Rheumatic afflictions, colds, fevers and convulsions; it diminishes trauma, promotes circulation, removes turbidity and filth, is anti-fungal, kills intestinal parasites, diminishes swelling, to include pain and swelling of the chest, internal and external trauma and dermatitis."

<u>PHARMACOPOEIA OF THE UNITED STATES OF AMERICA</u>

1947, 13th Revision, page 103-105

Extensive references appear in this formulary well before the 8th Edition published in May of 1900, specifically identifying this injectable substance at 200 ml intramuscular to be within normal limits.

GOODMAN and GILLMAN PHARMACOLOGICAL BASIS OF THERAPEUTICS

7th Edition, page 952; uses include internal, external and dentistry.

MARTINDALE INTERNATIONAL PHARMACOPOEIA

29th Edition, 1989-page 1552

References here are again extensive to include camphor as an injectable by subcutaneous or intramuscular means, for treatment of respiratory ailments and as adjunct for dispersion of gall stones.

The 1994 Canadian Investigational and Emergency Drug List includes 714X for Anti-Cancer and Immune Related Disease Therapy. (Drug Information Center, Ontario College of Pharmacists, Toronto, Canada.)

PROTOCOL FOR USING 7 1 4 X

Composition: Trimethylbicyclonitr amino heptane Cl, 714X,

Range of application: 714X is referred to as an immune function stabilizer or a pro-biotic life force potentiator and can be effective in treating degenerative, viral and immuno-deficient diseases.

Contra-indications: None known.

Side-effects: Since January of 1990 over 1,000 patrons in Canada under the Emergency Drug Relief Act are working with over 430 doctors who have issued over 4,500 patient applications for 714X with no reported side-effects.

Length of Treatment: The duration of treatment is determined by individual case and may range in length from two months to two years. In the case of cancer six months is the recommended minimum treatment period. After each series of twenty-one daily injections, the treatment may be continued without interruption or may be stopped for three days.

Interaction with other drugs:

1. Vitamins E and B-12 should not be used with 714X. B-12 augments cell proliferation and E creates a sheath around the cancer cell protecting it from the immune system.

2. Morphine: Morphine (or any opium derivative) is a powerful immune function blocker. It is advisable that the use of

morphine be gradually reduced to nil during 714X treatment within 15 days or as early as is tolerable.

Mode of Administration: There are three modes of administration:

1. The most effective and primary method is either intra or peri-nodular injection (see injection instructions).

2. The secondary is by Ultrasonic nebulization.

3. Sublingual drops (effective in cases of herpes and viral cold and flu infections, but not indicated for treating degenerative or immuno-deficient disease as the 714X enters the blood not the lymphatic system).

Dosage:

10 series of 21 consecutive daily injections is required for a minimum period of 6 months in cases of cancer. For other circumstances treatment may last from 2 months to 2 years according to the need of the patient. If the patient is thought to be terminal then the 714X may be taken once by injection and a second time per day by ultrasonic nebulization.

Recommended dosages

1st day - intra or peri-nodular injection of 0.10 cc

2nd day - intra or peri-nodular injection of 0.20 cc

3rd day - intra or peri-nodular injection of 0.30 cc

4th day - intra or peri-nodular injection of 0.40 cc

5th day and on - intra or peri-nodular injection of 0.50 cc each.

Begin and maintain each subsequent cycle at 0.5 cc

N.B. The determination of dosage levels is based on seventeen years of empirical studies. Case history failures have in some cases been the consequence of not following the protocol.

Pediatric Dosage:

Child's dosage may depend on size and weight. However, in most cases the above protocol is followed to the 0.3 cc dosage level and maintained at that amount.

Storage: 714X must be refrigerated once in use. The product must not be exposed to ultra-violet light, and otherwise has an indefinite shelf life.

IMPORTANT DIETARY RECOMMENDATIONS

Thousands of studies have been completed showing the amazing health benefits of a PLANT-BASED-DIET.

Live a longer, healthier life with the people you love.
After transitioning to a whole food, plant-based lifestyle, you will likely experience improved sleep and energy, decreased weight, and an overall sense of wellness.
But you may also lower your risk of heart disease, diabetes, and cancer.

Lower Risk of HEART DISEASE

Fact: About one of every three deaths in the U.S. results from heart disease, stroke and other cardiovascular diseases.

In Dr. Dean Ornish's well known Lifestyle Heart Trial, patients following a low-fat vegetarian diet had the following results after one year:

Chest pain began to disappear within weeks of starting program.

Average LDL (bad cholesterol) dropped from 152 mg/dL to 95 mg/dL

82% of patient's angiograms showed arteries reopening

Dr. Caldwell Esselstyn studied 23 Cleveland Clinic patients studied 23 Cleveland clinic patrons who had severe coronary artery disease (combined 49 cardiac events). The 17 patients following a plant-based diet for the duration of the study had the following results:

Angiograms showed opening of coronary arteries

All reduced their total cholesterol to lower than 150 mg/dL

No additional cardiac events

Lower Risk of DIABETES

Fact: In the U.S., 29.1 million people have diabetes (about 10% of the population). If current trends continue, one in three adults could have diabetes by 2050.

James Anderson, M.D. studied a group of Type 1 & 2 diabetic patrons following a mostly plant-based diet, all of whom had been taking insulin prior to their dietary change. Here are the results after three weeks:

Type 1 diabetic patients reduced their medication on average by 40% and 24 of the 25 Type 2 diabetic patients were able to discontinue their insulin

A recent study from the Harvard T.H. Chan School of Public Health surveyed 200,000 health professionals for more than 20 years and found that those following a healthy plant-based diet had a 34% lower risk of developing diabetes

Lower Risk of CANCER

Fact: Approximately 39% percent of men and women will be diagnosed with cancer of any type at some point during their lifetime. A large prospective study found that the occurrence of all cancers were lower for those eating a plant-based diet as compared to those eating the Standard American Diet.

A study that looked at men and women between the ages of 50 to 65 found that those eating higher protein diets had a 75% increase in overall mortality and four-fold increased risk of dying from cancer.

The American Cancer Society (February 13, 2015) published their recommendations that cancer survivors should follow plant-based diets that are high in fruits, vegetables and

Medical and nutritional programs should always be based on a thorough understanding by the patron and active consultation with the 'attending physician.

IT IS RECOMMENDED YOU DO INCLUDE IN YOUR DIET:

- Veal and corn-fed chicken,
- Broiled, boiled (fish curry is excellent) or baked flat fish; or
- Flat fish cooked without oil (flounder, halibut, turbot, sole, orange roughy, fruits and vegetables
- Juice from FRESH fruits and vegetables.

- (Fresh juice is absorbed up to 80% by the intestinal walls and may provide the mineral salts, vitamins and sugars needed for metabolism.)

DO DRINK:

One to three liters per day of uncarbonated mineral water to benefit and assist the kidneys and liver.

IT IS RECOMMENDED YOU DO NOT EAT:

- Beef or Pork (most are injected with antibiotics just prior to slaughter.) White flour or refined flour
- Food colorings or preservatives Artificial flavorings
- Coffee, tea, alcohol or chocolate Fried foods
- Dairy products, i.e. milk, cream, butter, yogurt or fermented cheeses
- Use stainless steel or glass cookware, avoiding in particular Teflon and aluminum.

There are numerous books on the topic of diet in relation to cancer patients and we are not attempting to address this vast subject here. However, it is considered important in the overall well-being and restoration of health.

The above are general recommendations to be used as a guideline to complement by diet a positive mental and vital approach to improving health and promoting ease, in the place of dis- ease. If you are already following an intelligent, balanced diet the correct protocol is to continue with the above recommendations in mind.

A product called Citricidal, which is non-toxic and anti-bacterial, is recommended to remove toxins from the skins of vegetables or fruit.

Please watch these videos for suggested dietary research and clarity.

PlantPure Nation - MUST SEE Documentary

https://youtu.be/A_i_vp9Vfho

Forks Over Knives: https://youtu.be/IrWb7wZ7MIU

Lymphatic System

Lymph and the lymphatic system: Of all our body systems, perhaps the most Ignored is the lymphatic system, although it forms a vast network throughout our body.

Lymph is a whitish fluid that is derived from blood plasma. As plasma circulates through the body, through the blood vessels and capillaries; the body is created to allow the lymph to pass through their walls. This is extremely beneficial to the health of the tissues because this provides the liquid environment essential for their survival.

The lymph moves through the vessels of the lymphatic system carrying away from the tissues dead cells and potentially harmful bacteria and viruses as well as cancer cells. At various points along the network, the vessels enlarge into small organ structures called lymph nodes (sometimes called lymph glands). Lymph nodes are thought to be the manufacturing sites of lymphocytes.

Swollen glands are actually swollen lymph nodes, where a battalion of lymphocytes is defending the body. Those in the neck, groin and armpits frequently exhibit the pain and swelling that may accompany and immune defense reaction.

The lymph in its effort to defend the body may inadvertently carry cancer cells throughout the body thus depositing cancer cells unwittingly in various other lymph nodes and organs. This is commonly referred to as metastasis. (see Naessens' discussion of the

CKF factor and Warburg discussion of the HCG secretion by cancer cells thus blocking the body's ability to recognize the cancer cells.)

The following pictures are the best available medical depiction and as such are not absolutely accurate.

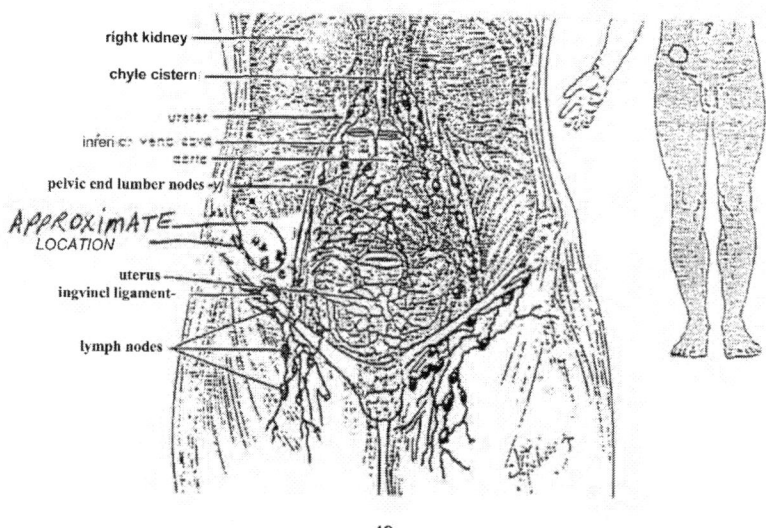

INJECTION TECHNIQUE

This procedure is intended to assist the medical professional and the patron's consultation with his doctor. It requires supervision and instruction to begin, but after learning the technique most patrons inject themselves or are assisted by a close friend, family member or visiting nurse.

714X is always administered by intra or peri-nodular injection into the right inguinal lymph nodes unless they have been surgically removed.

If the lymph node is hard, swollen or affected directly by the disease do not inject directly into the lymph but into the surrounding area whence it will be absorbed by the matrix into the lymphatic system.

The recommended needle is 27 Gauge x 3/8 inch. However, some patrons find the 28-gauge 1/2 inch preferable to their physical form. The syringes are calibrated in tenths of cubic centimeters, cc's, to facilitate exact measurement of 714X to be injected, or used for nebulization.

Prescription requirements for syringes vary from state to state, however for reference the syringe commonly used is B-D 305542 for the 27-gauge x 3/8 inch.

1) The patron is in a comfortable position lying on his back. An ice-pack, wrapped in a single sheet of paper towel, is placed on

the right inguinal-area injection site (see picture) for 10- 15 minutes.

2) Since time is required (approximately 12 to 15 minutes when 0.5 cc are given) the person making the injection should place himself in a chair in a position so as to make his arm comfortable while injecting.

3) Briefly clean the injection site, preferably with 90% ethyl alcohol if available. If ethyl is not available then you must allow the area to evaporate before the injection. Point the short injection-needle at approximately a 45-degree angle to the horizontal body with the needle pointing toward the right shoulder and the plunger toward the right foot. If an excessively painful burning persists you may be in the muscle and need to move the injection site toward the soft tissue.

4) Inject very slowly (12 to 15 minutes for .5 ml). Introduction of the 714X into the lymphatic system requires patience and skill. Too rapid an injection of even a small amount may create a sharp burning sensation. 714X is well tolerated and has no side effects.

5) When you have finished the injection and removed the needle, place an ice pack again over the injection site for about 12-15 minutes after the injection.

6) Finally, the patient should rest for about 15-20 minutes after the injection. A good time for this process is the early morning when vital function is on the rise.

DeVilbiss AeroSonic™ Ultrasonic Nebulizer

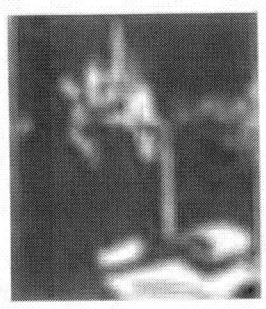

The AeroSonic operates on a "patient demand1* system of delivery; i.e., aerosol remains in the chamber until it is in- haled. After 30 seconds of operation, AeroSonic will automatically turn itself off. This designed- in feature lets you walk away or take care of other tasks without wasting or overheating expensive medication. To continue, simply press the button for another 30 seconds of therapy, AeroSonic from DeVilbiss—puts you in control of your aerosol therapy!

Specifications

Size	5" x 5.25" x 2.25* (13cm x 13cm x 6cm)
Weight	2.5 lbs.' (1.1 kg)
Sound Level	0 UBA
Electrical Requirements	120VAC, 60Hz, 12VDC, 900mA (Model 5000D) 220-240VAC, 50Hz, 12VDC, 900mA (Model 50001)
Operating Power	11 watts maximum

Consumption	
Frequency	2.25 MHz
Nebulization Rate	0.3ml/minute minimum
Particle Size Range	1-3 microns
MMAD	1.8 microns
Nebulizer Capacity	9 ml
Battery Running Time	45 minutes maximum
Battery Recharge Time	12 hours from fully discharged battery
Warranty	2 years; battery' 90 days

★ *Controlling unit and chamber weigh! only; does no! include accessories.*

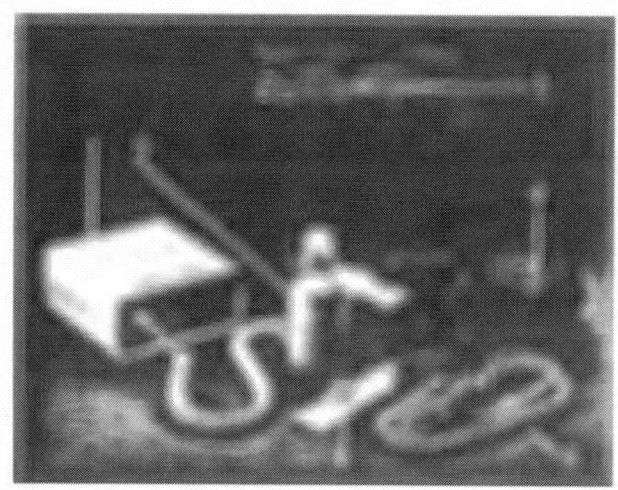

AeroSonic Model 5000D/5000I ultrasonic nebulizer includes:

1) Controlling Unit

2) Chamber Assembly

3) Carrying Case

4) AC to DC Adapter/Charger

5) Negative-Ground DC Power Cord

6) Mouthpiece with Check Valve & Adapter

Accessory/Replacement Items

5000D-641 Chamber Dome & Mouthpiece(6/package)
5000D-642 Medication Chamber (1 each)
5000D-643 AC to DC Adapter/Charger 120Vt 60 Hz (1 each)
50001-643 AC to DC Adapter/Charger 220/240V, 50 Hz (1 each)
5000D-644 Carrying Case (1 each)
5000D-645 Negative-Ground DC Power Cord (I each)
5000D-646 Positive-Ground DC Power Cord (1 each)
8500D-608 Safe-Vent Exhalation Filter, Mouthpiece & One-way Valve (20/case)
8500D-609 Mouthpiece with Check Valve & Adapter (6/package)
580AM Standard-Range Pulmo-Graph Peak Flow Monitor (12/case)
580PM Low-Range Pulmo-Graph Peak Flow Monitor (12/case)

THE PROTOCOL FOR THE USE OF AN ULTRASONIC NEBULIZER For SOMATO-THERAPY With 714X

Dosages in this protocol are for an adult: 0.5 cc 714X and 0.5 cc Sodium Chloride Solution .9% injectable, (do not use a brand that is mixed with isopropyl alcohol).

Inhalation Instructions

1. Aspirate: withdraw exactly 0.5 ml out of the usual 6.0 ml vial of 714X, by using the same type syringe and needle, as is used for injection, Allergy - or skin testing type syringe with 27 x 3/8" needle, spray this small amount of solution directly towards the golden spot in the center of your cone-shaped De Vilbiss ultrasound nebulizer inhalation unit.

2. Now aspirate again 0.5 ml out of your red plastic vial containing Sodium Chloride solution, using the same syringe with attached needle. You may have to use caution in holding this vial horizontally, while aspirating the solution. (Since this plastic vial contains 3.0 ml, it is good for 6 treatment-mixes. Store the opened vial vertically in a small glass and place it in your refrigerator.)

3. After you have sprayed the 0.5 ml Sodium Chloride solution into your inhalation unit - just like you did with 714X solution both solutions mix instantly, apply the plastic dome to your hand- held unit and apply one of your two mouthpieces to the dome.'

4. You are now ready for your inhalation therapy. **Please make sure you read the De Vilbiss "Aerosonic" nebulizer unit instruction booklet prior to your first inhalation.** The battery unit has to be charged at least 16 hours prior to first use. You can leave your battery unit on "charge" (yellow light - ON) during treatment cycles.

5. By pushing the -ON- switch at the battery unit, you will notice two green lights come on. A fine mist will be instantly forming within your nebulization chamber, easily visible through your plastic dome. After 30 seconds, the unit will turn itself off. For

your second activation and all thereafter, push the green button at the hand-held nebulizer unit; follow instruction manual guidelines.

6. It is recommended to exhale, prior to inhaling with a slow, deep breath for your first 714X inhalation. Hold your breath a few seconds, before exhaling. You may also do so continuously until all solution is gone, or you can take one deep breath at a time in intervals. The unit will always shut itself off after approximately 30 seconds (to prevent overheating of ultrasound unit).

7. If you can, allow a rest period of 20 to 30 minutes after each inhalation treatment.

8. Never submerge hand-held inhalation unit totally in cleaning solution. Follow cleaning instructions as per De Vilbiss instruction manual.

In response to inquiries: only an ULTRASOUND-type inhalation system can provide the ultra-fine mist that is necessary to reach even the smallest branch and ramification of your bronchial "tree" and therefore the large surface lymphatic "lining" of your lungs. Older units (like table models with long rubber hoses - as seen on the video) lose too much substance and are not recommended for treatment anymore. The "DeVilbiss Aerosonic Ultrasonic Nebulizer"™ is the best on the market today and it is considerably smaller, portable, re-chargeable and much easier to use than the older models.

Do not re-use the residue. Clean the capsule after each use with a cotton swab.

Introducing the most highly calibrated Cancer-Profile and Immune-Spectrum Blood Test

simple questions, concrete answers by

Dietmar Schildwaechter, M.D., Ph.D. Chief Medical Investigator

How can I know for sure if I have cancer?

How will I know if I am improving during treatment?

"Is there a reliable scientific test that tells me whether I have no cancer risk right now and can this test tell me whether I am out of danger? *

Yes, this is one of the features of this test. If anyone in your family had or has cancer, statistically increasing cancer risk, all relatives can benefit from this test.

"What about the cancer patient who was diagnosed some time ago, had perhaps Surgery or Chemotherapy or Radiation, or any combination and was told that he is free of cancer. Is he really ok? *

They may be, but no Scan, or MRI, or X-ray can tell for sure. These tests measure a "status quo" at the time they were taken. They never really tell of all-important functional dynamics and whether an individual still has existing primary cancer activity, new flare-up or metastatic activity and tendency for cancer to spread to other organs until a recurrence is finally determined by a doctor.

"Can this test tell me the real situation, whether I am out of danger, or whether there still is activity so I can do something about bringing it under control? *

Absolutely, this is yet another feature of this highly calibrated test.

"My doctor told me I am in remission. What does this mean? *

An individual with cancer, regardless at what stage of disease, is in remission when there is no primary and no metastatic activity and definitely no more progression of disease. This test profile with its sophisticated calibration can ascertain when you are in remission and out of danger.

I am and/or was treated with toxic therapies that severely depressed my immune-system. Can this test tell me what the status of my immune-system is at this time? *

Yes. Your immune-profile is a very important part of this test. We are now aware of the importance of our immune-system and the role it plays in protecting us from disease. The interpretation of your test results will tell you where you stand with your immune-defense situation at this time.

If I do have a risk to develop cancer within a period of one to two years can I reverse this risk?

Yes, if your immune system is low, we can recommend the necessary steps to strengthen it. In 1977 scientists established with statistically significant correlation that cancer is a preventable disease.

"Why was this important finding suppressed? *

The answer may lie in the documentable fact that cancer is one of the highest profit-makers for pharmaceutical giants and institutional medicine.

Dietmar Schildwaechter, M.D., Ph. D, of Sovereign Consultants, International and Chief Medical Investigator of this project, brings thirty-six years of knowledge and expertise in preventive medicine, early cancer detection, therapy response and guidance to the individual interpretation of each test result.

Cancer and Immune Profile Test

In order to establish a baseline of health and to track progress through the treatment process, a blood test is available which will indicate the presence of primary and metastatic cancer activity, liver function and immune function.

This blood test identifies and quantifies in a highly calibrated, manually conducted test five significant markers, the HCG (human chorionic gonadotropic hormone) by the HCG-beta- chain test, PHI (phosphohexose isomerase), the key enzyme in glycolysis which is greatly increased in cancer cell lines, GGTP for liver function, CEA (carcinoembryonic antigen) and DHEA-S.

The FDA requires an adequate means to monitor and track progression or regression during clinical use of an unapproved substance within the scope of the Institutional Review Board. Beyond these requirements the test allows the following:

A. For Prevention of disease:

   1. Establish an individual's health baseline.
   2. Determine an individual's immune defense status.

B. In established disease:

   1. Determine activity status, such as primary and secondary in malignant diseases not possible with status quo type scans or MRIs, thus allowing:

2. Exact monitoring of response to whatever treatment chosen by treating physician and/or patron, conventional as well as unconventional.

3. permits exact and scientific determination of remission in a patron.

4. Establishes cures over longer period interval testing.

5. Thus, preventing recurrence or relapse of disease.

C. For Scientific Clinical Studies and Trials

1. Eliminates double blind etc., studies with high degree of inaccuracies (certainly from a true epidemiological scrutiny).

2. Eliminates randomized trials.

3. Provides early risk factors for malignancies as a true prevention, therefore, complements cancer-search at too late a (clinical) stage with reduced survival chances (Mammography, Colonoscopy, etc.).

4. Provides exact clinical-biochemical parameter results for effectiveness of new substances.

D. In conjunction with unconventional medical practices.

1. Complements Gaston Naessens' Somatoscopic diagnosis

2. Monitors effect of Cell-Milieu-Medicine, fetal tissue therapy, bio-electronic and homeopathic approaches.

DHEA-S

(De-Hydro-Epi-Androsteron)

Dr. Nieper compares the immune system with the army (which calls out the reserves when there is danger), and the anti-cancer surveillance system with the police whose strength is essentially fixed.

The latter system includes mechanisms for gene repair, and certain steroids such as tumosteron and DHEA. Approximately 60% of all people have sufficient DHEA in their blood to be protected from cancer. Of the remaining 40% about half will develop hidden cancer but not die from it while the rest (20%) will die of diagnosed cancer.

A lack of DHEA has been correlated with peculiarities of the person's character -- non aggressive, amiable, easily depressed and indecisive.

DHEA-S is produced in the adrenal glands and circulates in the body as DHEA sulfate. A special activation factor, (which possibly is produced in the pineal gland or the thymus gland or the small intestines) changes DHEA-S into free DHEA.

DHEA paralyzes an enzyme (glucose-g-phosphate dehydrogenase) which is of primary importance to the action of cancer cells. This drastically reduces the vitality of the cancer cell and makes it possible for lymphocytes and other white blood cells to overcome the cancer cell.

Dr. Nieper found that during the course of disease, there is a tendency for the DHEA level to gradually decrease, sometimes to values less than 0.1 (100 nano-grams per milliliter). The cancer patient then does not have sufficient starting material to form free DHEA.

There are a number of drugs whose side effects are to cause the level of DHEA-S to drop. Most prominent are the clofibrates that are used to reduce lipid levels. A correlation has been found between higher cholesterol levels in the blood and lower frequency of cancer-if accompanied by higher values of DHEA.

DHEA was isolated by the German Nobelist Butenandt in 1934 and analyzed by the German chemist and Nobelist Windaus. However, the credit for having identified it as an important pillar of our anticancer surveillance system goes to Arthur Schwartz and his coworkers at Temple University in Philadelphia.

A summary of Dr. Hans Neiper's discussion of DHEA from "Revolution in Medicine and Health,"

November 1958.

HCG

(Human Chorionic Gonadotropic hormone)

Radioimmunoassay for the HCG-Beta-chain allows the quantitation of minute amounts of human choironic gonadotropic hormone even in the presence of LH, FSH and TSH. The obvious value is the detection of pregnancy within 2-3 days after conception, detection of micro abortion and detection and follow-up of HCG-secreting tumors.

Teratoma, hydatidiform mole and choriocarcinomas in the uterus, ovaries, testes, mediastinum, pineal and pituitary glands, stomach, lungs, esophagus and bladder have long been recognized as trophoblastic HCG-secreting tumors. However, HCG-B has been found in patients with practically all types of malignancies where trophoblasts were not expected:

1. testicular, non-trophoblastic gastrointestinal: carcinoid, colonic/rectal, gastric, pancreatic, small intestinal

2. hematopoietic: leukemia, all types of lymphomas, multiple myeloma, sarcomas: fibrosarcoma, leiomyosarcoma, osteogenic sarcoma.

3. miscellaneous tumors: breast, thyroid, uterine, bladder, adrenal gland, insulinomia, pheochromocytoma

4. lung carcinoma

5. hepatoma/hepatoblastoma.

Indeed, it seems that the HCG-secreting trophoblast may play an important role and it may be closely associated with not only embryogenesis but also carcinogenesis. As more data is becoming available, utilizing the sensitive and specific HCG-B test, it becomes evident that the frequency and types of tumors associated with HCG production are much greater than it has been suspected.

Due to the extreme sensitivity of the test (0.0025IU/ml or about 0.2 ng/ml) it is possible to detect, without localization, ongoing malignancies at a very early stage. Once a base level has been established, a patient's response to therapy can be monitored. The probability of detecting HCG in cancers of all types is, according to the literature surveyed, 10-100%. The longest interval for elevated HCG-B before cancer diagnosis was 26 months.

PHI

(Phospho-Hexose Isomerase or glucose phosphate isomerase)

PHI is a key enzyme in glycolysis, i.e. the main anaerobic energy generating step of glucose metabolism. Glycolysis has been observed to become greatly increased in cancer cell lines, hence the measuring of PHI became accepted as a valuable too! in the appraisal of neoplasias.

Elevated PHI levels were found in localized and metastasized cancers of the: bladder, bone, brain, breast, intestines, liver, lungs, lymphosarcoma, melanoma, mouth, head, neck, esophagus, pancreas, prostate, ovary, stomach, colon, rectum and uterus.

PHI has been shown to be elevated in more patients with neoplasia than other enzymes. However, it may not be elevated in the serum of some patients in an early state of neoplasia and indeed, it is not elevated in the serum of some patients with active diseased state. The detection of the enzyme at elevated levels may warrant a more thorough evaluation of the patient.

Once a base level has been established, PHI is a promising enzyme in following the effectiveness of therapy. When, for instance, this enzyme was monitored during treatment of breast cancer, changes in activity followed progression or regression of tumor growth and antedated other laboratory evidence by days or weeks.

It was also found to be indicative of regressions induced by steroids, radio-therapy, oophorectomy, chemotherapy, and hypophysectomy. In cases of confirmed malignancy any elevation or drop, even within the normal ranges, may be significant.

PHI may be elevated in heart, liver and skeletal muscle diseases. Preliminary data indicates that PHI levels parallel CEA results (Personal communications, Miami Heart Institute and Worthington Biochemical Corporation), however, it does not seem to be affected by smoking and it seems to reflect upon a greater variety of diseases. (The performance cost of PHI is about one-half of that of CEA.)

PHI is very abundant in the red blood cells: therefore, it is imperative that the serum specimen is free from hemolysis.

References for HCG:

B.D. Weintraub and S.W. Rosen, Ectopic Production of HCS and HGB by Non-trophoblastic Cancers. J. Clin. Endocr., 13, 94, 1971.

F. Civantos and A.M. Rywlin, Carcinomas with Trophoblastic Differentiation and Secretion of Chorionic Gonadotropins. Cancer, 29, 789, 1972.

G.D. Braunstein, et al., Ectopic Production of HCG by Neoplasms. Annals Int. Med., 78, 39, 1973.

A.S. Rabson et al., Production of HCG in vitro by a Cell Line Derived from a Carcinoma of the Lung. J. Natl. Cancer Inst., 50, 669, 1973.

W.S. Floyd and S.L. Cohn, Gonadotropin Producing Hepatoma. Obst. Gyn, 41, 665, 1973.

D.W. Gold et al., Gonadotropin-Secreting Renal Carcinoma. Cancer. 33, 1048, 1974.

D.P. Goldstein et al., The clinical Application of Specific RIA for HCG in Trophoblastic and Nontrophoblastic tumors. Surg, Gvnec. Obst., 138. 747, 1974.

D.C. Torney etal., Biological Markers in Breast Carcinoma. Cancer, 35, 1095, 1975.

R.R. Williams et al., Tumor-Associated Antigen Levels Antedating the Diagnosis of Cancer in the Framingham Study. J, Natl. Cancer Inst., 58, 1547, 1977.

References for PHI:

0. Bodansky, Serum PHI in Cancer: II. As an Index of Tumor Growth in Metastatic Carcinoma of the Breast. Cancer, 7, 1191, 1954.0. Bodansky, Serum PHI in Cancer: III. As an Index of Tumor Growth in Metastatic Carcinoma of the Prostate. Cancer, 8, 1087, 1955.

M.M. Griffith and J.C. Beck, The Value of Serum PHI as an Index of Metastatic Breast Carcinoma Activity. Cancer, 16, 1032. 1963/

M.H. Gault et al., Serum Enzymes in Patients with Carcinoma of the Lung. Canada Med. Assoc. J96,87. 1967.

C.R. Ratliff et al., Serum LDH, PHI and Serological Evidence of Malignant Diseases. Clin. Chem., 16, 527. 1970.

C.R. Ratliff, Serum PHI: A glycolytic Enzyme for Appraising Neoplasia. 4th Ann. So. Calif. Lab. Conference, Anaheim, March 6, 1973.

Worthington Biochemical Corporation, In Case of Malignancy-PHI Monitors Therapy, 1974.

Letter from Diet mar Schildwaechter, M.D. Ph.D. to Ms. Jeanne O'Hara, Medicare regarding reimbursement for Cancer-immune profile test.

Ms., Jeanne O'Hara
MEDICARE General Delivery
Department of Benefits - Physician's Services
P.O. Box 890089
Camphill. PA 17089-0089

March 13, 1995

Re: CA-Profile and Immune -Profile clinical-biochemical parameter testing (according to Schandl and Nieper) for Us patients.

Dear Ms. O'Hara,

Pursuant to our telephone discussion yesterday, April 19, 1994, I am herewith attaching to this letter a 1-page copy of my testimony at N.I.H., since it describes in a concise way the features of this test.

The problem appears to be an unwillingness, of even first-class laboratories, to go into the required, highly scientific calibration of our markers, so they become meaningful differential diagnostic values.

In today's automated systems, clinical pathologists who indicated an interest to work with us, after learning the extent of required, qualified personnel, time and financial involvement etc., remarked "This is impractical for use and perhaps questionable in its financial reward.

Since Dr. Emile K. Schandl, Ph.D., pioneered this profile in combining biostatistically-overlapping markers to achieve an unsurpassed accuracy in 1977 {duly published and presented at scientific meetings), it has become the only reliable and constantly upgraded functional monitoring test. Our high-cost (certainly for insurance carriers) Scans, MRIs, or tomograms, etc. are strictly "status quo" examinations, not giving us any clue as to the functional dynamics of primary or metastatic activity, when patients are truly in "remission" how their immune-defense situation is, etc. Recent, MAYO-clinic initial source negative criticism about the value of CEA-markers* as a single monitoring test for Colon Cancer patients is a confirmation of our experience that it is very limited as a SINGLE marker!

In regard to insurance re-imbursement and payments for these profile tests, let me state that there apparently has been no problem (except with KAISER or HMO). AH tests have the basic Blue Cross code number. Even European socialized medical insurance systems do re-imburse patients. Most tests are ordered by their physicians.

Samples from the U.S. and Canada are shipped daily to Germany by international air carriers. The results are being faxed to us and accordingly interpreted. The interpretation for all tests regardless from what country and whether for patients directly, referring physicians, clinics or hospitals, are done by me.

The German laboratory is one of the leading fully licensed and high caliber laboratories in Europe, my association goes back to the early seventies (70s) while I was Medical Director of the newest Cancer

Rehabilitation Hospital within the German Government's social medical system. I am still a licensed physician within the European community, but retired from the practice of medicine in the United States. Sovereign Consultants International was founded thereafter and is a Loudoun County, Virginia licensed and registered firm.

Laboratory super-bills are similar to the one's used for procedures previously. They reflect the higher cost for sophisticated calibration methods required for accuracy and meaningful interpretation.

I hope this letter will help to establish a baseline for-at least partial reimbursement for patients like Mrs. Thank you for your courtesy and cooperation.

Very truly yours,

Dietmar Schildwaechter, Ph.D., M.D.

Enzyme Therapy of Cancer by Max Wolf, M.D.

Proteolytic enzymes in the treatment of malignant tumors have been used in historical times already. Long before the discovery of America by Columbus, medicine men of the Indians applied fruits and leaves of the papaya plant to malignant tumors, they used local enzyme therapy empirically. It was known that fresh papaya fruits favorably influenced inflammations and edemas, that wounds, burns, bruises or infections healed faster and pains subsided sooner, also that malignant tumors responded sometimes to this therapy.

About the year 1820, Physick in Philadelphia was the first to use proteolytic enzymes in the form of stomach juice for surface cancer with good results. In 1836 Schwann isolated pepsin from stomach juice, in 1871 Purden and in 1888 Douglass applied the enzyme pepsin to ulcerated cancerous lesions. At the end of the 19th century the first attempts were made to give pepsin intramuscular and trypsin intravenous.

In the year 1902 the enzyme therapy of cancer received a decided impulse when John Beard began cancer treatment with enzyme extracts of the pancreas. His therapeutic successes caused great excitement.

By 1906 he had used trypsin, amylopsin and other unknown enzymes of the pancreas in treating different cancers. His comprehensive book: The Enzyme treatment of Cancer stirred up great interest among many scientists and clinicians who soon went about to develop further this therapy and to use it extensively.

Beard, the leading embryologist of his time, concluded from his studies for many years of the embryonal development of animals that during the progressive differentiation of the developing organs undifferentiated polyvalent "sex" cells wander from the trophoblast mainly through the mesoderm within the embryo to their goal of destination, the gonads.

Countless cells of them get stuck on this voyage between somatic cell aggregates.

These everywhere dispersed embryonal trophoblast isles remain dormant, according to Beard, and do not multiply during the entire life span of the individual.

However, the one or the other cell can by specific irritants, cancerogens, start a cell division and thus form a functionless tissue island, a tumor, indeed, American scientists, like Hayflick, during recent years were able to identify in tissue cultures of the different organs such scattered cells, about 0.25 to 0.5% of the total, the least number in heart tissues.

They differ morphologically from the other cells by absorbing more dyestuff, but without mutagenic or cancerogenic irritations they remain dormant. When their mitosis starts, they stain darker than the somatic cells, also typical characteristics of tumor cells appear. Compared with normal cells, they are potentially immortal, i.e. they multiply without any restraint through hundreds of subcultures while all somatic cells in the cultures "age", they lose their ability to further divide and die after not more than 50 mitoses.

Soon physicians all over the world were interested in the theoretical as well as the excellent therapeutic results. The preparations used consisted mainly of freshly prepared pancreatic extracts, Campbell, Goeth, Duprey, Curtfield, Marsden, Meggit, Cleaves, Shaw-McKenzie, Little, Bainbridge.

Hald, Pusey and Blumenthal reported before that intra-tumoral Injections of trypsin would bring about a relatively fast softening of the tumor, with aseptic liquefaction. However, besides the therapeutic successes also side effects of a pyrogenic and toxic nature appeared.

Finally, they began to produce pancreas extract industrially for a longer shelf life of the product. But it was unknown at that time that after a few hours of storing at room temperature the enzyme activity of the liquid extracts was lost. Their use resulted in a deterioration of therapeutic results obtained and led finally to the fact that the enzyme therapy of cancer was forgotten, or rather fell into hibernation.

Only much later the factors were recognized which ruined the confidence in Beard's therapeutic development: the instability of the enzyme products, their antigenicity and the impurity of the extracts used that time as well as their contents of pyrogens and toxic admixtures.

When much later it became possible to produce crystalline and pure enzymes, the therapeutic application could be resumed again in larger amounts. Sumner crystallized in 1926 Urease, Northrop in 1930 Pepsin, Northrop and Kunitz, Trypsin. Thus, it became possible to stabilize the enzymes and to eliminate pyrogens and other toxic substances.

In 1934 in Vienna Freund discovered that in the serum of people or animals free of cancer chemical substances existed which were able to dissolve cancer cells, while the blood of cancer patients was lacking this ability.

Besides that, the Freund-Kaminer team also found that the serum and urine of cancer patients not only was lacking in cancerolytic property but that cancer cells were even protected by it against dissolution by normal serum and produce a cancer-protection substance in the serum.

If, for instance, to normal serum half the amount of cancer serum is added, the former loses its proteolytic capacity against cancer cells. Freund isolated this water-soluble, thermolabile substance from the serum and urine of men and horses free of cancer; he called it "Normal Substance" and used it with partly good results as parenteral therapy on inoperable cancer cases.

Furthermore, this phenomenon led to the development of the Freund-Kaminer reaction.

This test indicated that the serum of cancer-free people and animals dissolves a large percentage of cancer cells in a fresh cancer suspension (later he used for this test heat-killed necrotic cells) or it changed them markedly.

However, cancer serum hardly affected them, it even protected them against disintegration by normal serum. Kretz and Benda could verify these facts, also Klein and Lustig. Freund had found 30 years earlier that cancer serum possesses these cancer- protective qualities which are derived from abnormal fatty acids found in the intestinal tract.

His directions to fight the cancer disease by diet (total elimination of animal fats and fermentative foods and by elimination, as much as possible, of the "abnormal," acid-fast, coli bacteria, which live in the colon of cancer patients, by "intestinal antiseptics" like menthol, or by enemas) are based upon these investigations.

Freund and Lustig showed in 1993 on tar cancers of mice that a cancerophile diet hastens the tumor development and the animals died earlier, while a cancerophile diet protects 50% of the mice.

On account of the beginning World War, Freund and Kaminer were forced to discontinue their activity in Vienna and therefore had no chance anymore to identify chemically the isolated Normal Substance. By Christiani in Vienna it was later identified as a cytolytic enzyme and, independently shortly before, by us (Wolf) as a proteolytic-lipolytic enzyme.

Christiani worked on the problem of closer examination of the cancerolytic enzymes and could demonstrate that the "normal substance" is in fact a hydrolytic enzyme which he called "solving enzyme". He proved 1938 that this solving enzyme is bound to the albumin fractions and is thermolabile.

It is present in the serum and urine of healthy people and animals (horses), but absent in the serum and urine of cancer patients. Later on, Christiani found in the serum of cancer patients some of the inhibitors of the solving enzyme.

They protect cancer cells against the solving enzyme and are produced by the cancer cells. Also, Freund knew about such inhibitors which were named "protective substances".

Cholesterol esters, e.g. cholesterol-butyrate or cholesterol-succinate have this protective action and indeed are identical with those formed by the cancer cells.

Christiani also could show that inhibitors, identified by him, could themselves be inactivated by a number of substances, like oxydation products of ergosterol or the 7- dehydrocholesterol. Such substances have acidic character: He called them deactivators. In vitro they were able to prevent the attachment of the inhibitor-the protection of the cancer ceil-to the solving enzyme, as well as to free again an already blocked enzyme.

Further investigations proved that the de-activator present in healthy people is bound to the globulin fraction of the serum. The de-activator is synthesized from 7-dehydrocholesterol by means of the enzyme ergosteroloxydase, which cannot bp demonstrated in cancer tissues.

Since then numerous scientists were able to prove that the serum of healthy men and animals is rich in proteolytic, lypolytic and amylolytic enzymes. Patients with more or less active inflammations or infections have in general a lower enzyme potential, but by far the lowest enzyme content as a rule is found in cancer cases (32,33).

Since in precancerous and in earliest stages of beginning cancers the enzyme niveau in the serum appears very reduced, it seems most probable that low enzyme values represent a predisposition or condition for the malignant process. Sometimes the low level is inherited, in some cases it may be caused by chronic infections, damage to the pancreas or other diseases, possibly also faulty nutrition.

Gaschler et al. determined the proteolytic activity in the serum of a great number of people. They found that healthy men in general have a high protease index, while this was reduced with sick people, particularly patients with chronic inflammations or infections, also in old age. The serum of cancer patients, of those with precanceroses and patients who later developed malignancies showed a significantly decreased proteolytic enzyme level.

The Gaschler test is very simple. It is not dependable, but in our experience with over 1000 tests, it gave some valuable information, particularly as a negative exclusion test for malignancies.

It was clinically applied that time to cancer patients with tumors of all different types, even in advanced stages. With the oral application of his enzyme mixture Gaschler could accomplish only some slight local beneficial effects. Therefore, he confined his therapy exclusively to parenteral application.

In several clinics of the Charite in Berlin, encouraging results were accomplished.

Elevation of general well-being, improved appetite, gain in weight and other subjective improvements were registered. With a number of patient's regressions could be determined.

All these results were taken in consideration during our own developments and experiments. We developed in numerous animal experiments and trials at the Biological Research Institute in N.Y. individual enzymes and enzyme combinations with and without activators which had selectively a lytic action on cancer cells.

In the experimental groups, on the other hand, the following events could be observed: first the cancer cells grew without restraint into all directions, fastest in the direction against the normal tissue. Almost suddenly the cancer cells stopped growing further.

They changed partly into a spindle shape, also ball-like form, some shriveled, became enucleated and finally dissolved, while the normal tissues showed hardly any influence by the enzymes added to the cultures. They rather pushed back the front rows of the tumor cells. The cell damages were much more pronounced than those seen in damage to normal tissues observed in the controls.

These characteristic pictures of cell cultures show the reaction of normal and malignant cells under influence by proteolytic enzymes.

While fibroblasts remain uninfluenced, cancer tissue undergoes lysis after a short period of time.

The enzymes tested in these experimental groups were solutions of trypsin, chymotrypsin, plasmin, kathepsin, pepsin, liver catalase, papain, ficin, bromelin, and enzyme extracts of lens esculenta, pisum sativum, aspergillus oryzae, spleen, thymus (mainly nucleases), liver and primarily the enzyme combination finally determined by us as optimal. *

During our investigation it was necessary to develop new tests for assaying the proteolytic and fibrinolytic activity in body fluids. The specificity and sensibility of the plate tests were not high enough; methods after Astrup and Mullertz.

In extensive animal experiments on rats we tested the proteolytic activity of the serum after taking the proteolytic enzymes mixture. It was given to the animals in gradually increasing amounts orally, intramuscular, intraperitoneal or by rectum. After 90 minutes the proteolytic activity of the serum was determined by the plate method mentioned. A significant relation between the proteolytic potential and the concentration of the enzyme mixture given was shown.

Some authors discuss the importance of general membrane defects in cancer. (Hoelzl-Wallach). They distinguish between:

1. plasma membrane (cell contact, cell surface, immunological changes),
2. mitochondrial membrane (protein and lipid synthesis),

3. lysosomal membrane,

4. nuclear membrane and

5. the endoplasmatic reticulum, responsible for enzymatic changes and enzyme biosynthesis

It concluded that the membrane hypothesis of tumors postulates that an oncogenic agent acts to introduce an inappropriate protein into or through cell membranes-either in replacement of or in addition to normal components.

'Proteolytic enzymes of fractionated hydrolysates of beef pancreas, calf thymus, pisum sativum, lens esculenta, papayotin, mannit.

Sagiroglu could show in his experiments that in stained malignant tissues many epithelioid cancer cells show smaller or larger membrane defects near the nucleus. Through these tears the cytoplasma leaked out producing the picture of a "nucleus halo" after staining. Such damages of the cell membrane of malignant cells could give a natural explanation for their selective destruction by enzymes.

Exact observations of the cancer cells made it probable that their cell membrane, in contrast to that of fibroblasts and other normal cells, is permeable for the proteolytic and lypolytic enzymes in our mixture. Thus, the catabolic enzymes penetrate into the inner cell and are able to dissolve the cytoplasma.

The fact that normal cells are more protected against lysis than cancer cells through enzyme inhibitors certainly also plays a part. But since the enzyme mixture used by us contains also lipolytic enzymes against which no inhibitors have been found so far, the cancer cell membrane seems to be insufficiently protected against these enzymes; a factor which therapeutically is very important.

All cell membranes consist mainly of phospholipids and mucopolysaccharides. They cannot normally be attacked by the specific enzymes present in small concentration in the blood, since no sufficiently wide pores exist which would allow the entrance of the macromolecules of the enzyme.

The protective cell wall becomes, however, penetrable for lytic enzymes when marked irritations lead to cell damages or to necrobiotic or necrotic processes. In such cases the penetration succeeds easily, also enzymes are set free from the lysosomes, thus bringing about an endogenous lysis.

Electron microscopic and isotopic investigations showed that catabolic enzymes penetrate also through membranes of malignant cells. Possibly this is brought about by the fact that the cell membrane shows defects and that it is incomplete during the rapid mitosis.

In further comprehensive experiments we investigated the effects of the enzyme combination besides in vitro tests, upon the different tumor implants, in rats and mice on chemically induced rat tumors and on spontaneous mamma carcinomas of dogs. The preparation Carzodelan® of Gaschler was part of in the investigations.

In both cases definite significant damages of the cancer cells could be demonstrated without influencing normal tissues.

The de-activator is present in all tissues except the thymus. With cancer patients this de-activator is not found in the tumor and in tumor-bearing organs, but in tumor-free organs in the form of a lactone. In this form it cannot de-activate the applied protective substance (inhibitor); it is biologically inert.

In the solid Ehrlich- carcinoma of the mouse, after intratumoral injection of Carzodelan® or of our mixtures, statistically significant tumor regression took place. The tumors partly ulcerated or necrotized, in other cases a partial shrinking in size appeared. Later on, the disease process leads to death but the prolongation of life was significant

During the examination of calf pancreas extract it was found that pure trypsin and chymotrypsin are to a great extent inhibited by the cancer serum, but their inhibition is blocked or is absent if amylases and lipase, but also certain other substances of the pancreas extraction are present.

The cytolytic effect of our enzyme mixture was demonstrated by animal experiments of several investigators. The enzymes administered via various routes to hamsters with cheek pouches of hetero-transplantable human tumors showed this anti-tumor effect; Goldenberg in personal communications.

One interesting model for the selective effect of proteolytic enzymes upon tumor cells is the spontaneous mamma adenoma of the sprague-Dawly rat. In all female animals of this certain strain a spontaneous fibroadenoma resp. adenofibroma develops in advancing age.

These tumors develop subcutaneously and can grow into all regions of the body.

They may reach a size twice the size of the whole rat. If the proteases are injected intratumorally in these rats, necrosis resp. liquefication of the tumor takes place till the entire tumor has disappeared. With tumors up to the size of a hen's egg, these results are always reproducible, with tumors beyond the size of a man's fist the success is not always constant.

As an explanation it may be mentioned that the tumor necrotises rapidly in rats and the death of the rat is caused by the overwhelming flooding's of the organism with the catabolic products of the tumor.

It is remarkable that the enzyme activity stops causing necroses as soon as all tumor tissue is dissolved, the surrounding healthy tissues (connective and. muscular tissues) are not affected. Also, the necrotized skin over the tumor heals during enzyme therapy without complications. Mostly not even noticeable scar tissue remains (Weigelt)

Especially clearly the protective effect of the enzyme mixture can be shown with the sarcoma 180 of the mouse. This sarcoma has a taking rate of over 95%. But in mice which received 4 days before and during transplantation 5 mg of the enzyme mixture, in only 20% of the animal's tumors were formed.

ENZYME THERAPY
by Kersten Schildwaechter

Enzyme therapy can be an important first step in staying healthy or restoring health- and well-being by helping to remedy digestive imbalances. Plant enzymes and pancreatic enzymes are used in complementary ways to improve digestion and absorption of essential nutrients. Treatment includes enzyme supplements, coupled with a healthy diet that features wholefoods.

For every chemical reaction that occurs in the body, enzymes provide the stimulus. "Enzymes are substances that make life possible," stated Edward Howell, M.D. who pioneered enzyme therapy in the United States. "No mineral, vitamin, or hormone can do any work without enzymes. They are the manual workers that build the body from proteins, carbohydrates, and fats. The body may have the raw building materials, but without the workers, it cannot begin!"

Both plant-derived and pancreatic enzymes are employed in enzyme therapy and they can be used independently or in combination. Plant enzymes are prescribed to enhance the body's vitality by strengthening the digestive system, while pancreatic enzymes are beneficial to both the digestive system and immune system. As proper digestive functioning is restored, many acute and chronic conditions may also be remedied.

Enzymes and Digestion

The human body makes approximately twenty-two different digestive enzymes, capable of digesting proteins, carbohydrates, sugars, and fats. People digest food in stages: beginning in the mouth, moving to the stomach, and finally through both small intestinal systems and the colon. At each step, specific enzymes break down different types of food. An enzyme designed to digest protein, for example, has no effect on starch. This process is balanced through acidity; each site along the digestive track has a different degree of acidity that allows certain enzymes to function while inhibiting others.

As enzymes begin digesting food in the mouth and continue their work in the stomach, plant enzymes derived from food itself or taken as a supplement also join in and become active. The food then enters the Duodenum, at the upper portion of the small intestine, where the pancreas, a sophisticated digestive organ that feeds enzymes into the gut, provides pancreatic enzymes to further break down the food. Final breakdown of remaining small molecules of food occurs in the Ileum, the lower part of the small intestine. Ideally, these enzymes can work together, digesting food and delivering nutrients to cells to maintain their health. Protocols in enzyme therapy are based on this sequence of events.

Plant Enzyme Therapy

As plant enzymes are essential for the proper digestion of food, they can play an important role in promoting good health. This is the basis of treatment in plant enzyme therapy. According to Howard F. Loomis, Jr., D.C., of Forsyth, Missouri, "The ability to absorb the nutrients in the food we eat is at the foundation of good health. If we treat digestive disorders, other complaints often clear up as a result. " In his own practice. Dr. Loomis tests his patients for enzyme deficiency and then replenishes this deficiency with enzyme supplements. Dr. Loomis adds, "Of course, if a patient is eating a diet of junk food, all the enzymes in the world won't improve bis or her basic health. Enzyme therapy needs to be combined with good eating habits. Fresh fruits, vegetables, nuts, and seeds can provide plentiful plant enzymes, and plant enzyme supplements are only meant to supplement those that naturally occur in food."

All four categories of plant enzymes have uses in plant enzyme therapy. Protease digests protein; amylase digests carbohydrates; lipase digests fat; and cellulase digests fiber. Plants are a person's only source of cellulase as the human body is unable to produce it. Numerous plant enzyme formulations on the market combine these enzymes.

Plant enzymes function in the stomach, predigesting the food, and plant enzyme therapy uses this to its advantage. This phenomenon was first proposed by Dr. Howell in the 1920s and the study of this process became his life's work. He stated, if the stomach is it As plant enzymes are essential for the proper digestion of food, they can play an important role in promoting good health., performing its proper role, and we are eating our foods well chewed and uncooked, a large portion of the intake will be partially digested before reacting with the stronger digestive juices found there. Moreover, fewer of your body's internal digestive enzymes will be called upon to perform the digestive function." It is this easing of the body enzymes' workload that is thought to contribute substantially to the healing effects of enzyme therapy. When the body receives plentiful supplies of enzymes, according to Dr. Howell, "most of its internal enzyme supplies are preserved for the important work of maintaining metabolic harmony." As a result, many body systems are strengthened.

This predigest ion of food happens during an interim period, before enough hydrochloric acid (HCI) accumulates in the stomach to begin the next stage in digestion, but this is not commonly known. As Lita Lee, Ph.D., of Eugene, Oregon, states, 'Many people don't believe this because they are told that gastric HCI excreted by the stomach destroys the enzymes.": Actually, it takes thirty to sixty minutes before enough HCI accumulates in the stomach to initiate the digestion of food. Further. HCI does not destroy these enzymes by making the environment more acidic. They are reactivated later in the duodenum, upper segment of the small intestine, Enzymes in die stomach can digest 30 to 40 percent of the starches we eat. And Dr, Lee adds, "By eating raw foods and taking food enzymes, 30 percent of the protein and 10 percent of the fat can be digested in the stomach in less than one hour."

Cooking food can destroy these important plant enzymes. They are more heat-sensitive than vitamins and are the first to be destroyed during cooking. They are destroyed by being heated above 118 degrees Fahrenheit, and, as Dr. Lee points out, "are deactivated or destroyed by pasteurizing, canning, and especially microwaving," However, while raw foods are recommended, a 100 percent raw foods diet is not necessary. Dr. Loomis points out that some people

may have problems digesting uncooked food because "Plant enzymes function in the of a lack of cellulase. "People who rarely eat raw foods, predigesting the food, food can have problems when they finally cat uncooked fruits and vegetables because they don't chew their food thoroughly," says Dr. Loomis. "Chewing liberates the cellulase out of the food, but when they eat the raw food and don't chew properly the cellulase is never released. Cellulase may also be lacking because of the way the food was handled by the suppliers. Some supermarket vegetables are missing cellulase because they have been sprayed with sulfites which can destroy these enzymes."
page 2 of 9

Plant Enzyme Deficiency

While inadequate nutritional and dietary intake has been considered by experts as the leading cause for enzyme deficiency and many resulting conditions such as frequent and repeated infectious diseases, we have to realize that food intake is an important factor, but not the only one. Our nutritional intake should be well balanced and not depend on cooked food alone, but should be vitamin rich with a lot of fresh vegetables and fresh fruits. However, a more important and usually overlooked factor is the detrimental administration of antibiotics. Sometimes antibiotics are administered over a very long period of time and sometimes repeatedly in short intervals and consisting of different types of antibiotic remedies to overcome the known development of resistance to antibiotic substances. In addition, the administration of cortisone not only by injection but also by topical application over various periods of time have a devastating effect on the intestinal system. Just as damaging is the application of antibiotics which for many patients dates back even to childhood and infancy.

Why is the application of antibiotics and cortisone damaging? The intestinal flora and predominantly E. coli are of utmost importance for proper digestion of carbohydrates, proteins, and fat. Its normal function and unharmed existence play an important part in the body's immune defense. situation. The unfortunate liberal use of antibiotics in our days, without establishing a "target" and performing the necessary culture and sensitivity testing, in every instance has a negative effect on the intestinal flora. Experienced researchers and clinicians in the field of micro-ecology found that patients with a history of antibiotics and / or cortisone showed tremendous deficiencies in their stool culture flora, sometimes to a total absence of E. coli. This was replaced by a pathological flora such as klebsiella or pseudomonas. If this situation exists, not only do many patients develop allergies and sometimes very severe reactions, but they no longer detoxify when food or water - polluted by chemicals or preservatives - is being taken. If patients in addition still have old mercury containing dental amalgam fillings (dark grey fillings used for filling cavities) that constantly, and during chewing, produce a microscopic abrasion, leading to a deposition of Mercury, the very sophisticated or perhaps very sensitive lymphatic lining of the intima (the inner lining of the small and large intestinal system) is paralyzed and is no longer able to detoxify.

If we are now supplying our enzymes as plant or animal enzymes (preferably in the proteolytic "Gaschler- Wolf formula*") a small dosage of enzymes such as one or two tablets only, would be deactivated by the toxic lining of the intima that is void of lymphatic activity. It therefore is of importance to supply these enzymes in a high enough dosage to certainly be beyond the deactivation threshold that exists in these patients. In other words, patients should be taking at least eight tablets upon rising in the morning and eight tablets upon retiring in the evening.

Why do we recommend the intake of these proteolytic enzymes as the first dosage in the morning and the last one at night? Proteolytic enzymes of the sophisticated Gaschler-Wolf, GW Formula may be partially deactivated by food protein. They should be taken at least half an hour before a meal at breakfast, or one hour after a meal at bedtime. Depending on the degree of immune deficiency, and a patient's susceptibility to all kinds of infectious diseases, preferably determined by the cancer and immune profile blood test, the dosage of these enzymes must be determined and then taken accordingly. If these important guidelines are not observed and the dosage of enzyme supplementation is neglected in perhaps too low a dosage, they cannot remove the toxins in the colon and cannot add to the necessary detoxification. Not only is food sometimes not properly digested but as stated earlier, toxins cannot be excreted. page 3 of 9

To support the enzyme supplementation for detoxification, the regeneration of a normal intestinal flora and reactivation of the lymphatic system of the intima, the natural production - especially of pancreatic enzymes - should be utilized. The pancreas, perhaps our most sophisticated organ, with a hormone producing part (insulin) and an enzyme producing portion, is activated just like other enzyme producing systems in the body by every food intake. By suggesting to clients with health problems to take repeatedly very small meals over the whole day, rather than adhere to three major meals, the pancreatic enzyme producing activity can be stimulated to a very high degree. Researchers have reported that the pancreas can produce up to four quarts of liquid enzymes. And in a unique metabolic system these pancreatic enzymes can be recycled. The more pancreatic enzymes are produced as a support of the proteolytic enzyme intake, the better off a patient will be.

In addition to the proteolytic enzyme formula and the stimulation of the body's own enzyme producing systems it is recommended to take superoxide dismutase, SOD enzymes as well as co-q-zyme, CoQ 10 enzymes, preferably combined, but separated from the proteolytic enzyme intake by a meal. In other words, while the proteolytic important enzymes should be taken after rising, before breakfast and 1 hour after dinner, at bedtime, the combination of a lower dosage of sod and co-q-zyme should be taken after breakfast and before dinner.

Benefits of Oxygen in Enzyme Therapy

The benefits of combined sod and co-q-zyme intake was mentioned in presentations of research papers at the Oxidative Medicine Association's annual convention in 1994 at Reston, Virginia. The combination of these two enzymes allows the body to produce its own hydrogen peroxide (H_2O_2). This additional oxygenation of the body again has a multiple role. The most important of it is to support a stimulation of the Immune System that is also being supported and restored by this combined enzyme supplementation. It should be noted that the immune system and especially the phagocytes and T-cells of the body's white blood cells require a lot of Oxygen (02) for their important activity. Dr. Otto Warburg and more recently Prof. Manfred Von Ardenne have proven the importance of Oxygen-multi step immuno-therapy, and it has been the backbone of biological Cancer-therapy in European countries for many years, including the GW-formula enzymes. Oxygen is utilized in many different forms. A lack of Oxygen and a depravation of 02 and reduction of angiogenesis like it is claimed as the effect of Shark Cartilage, and unavoidably paralyzes the body's immune defenses. Furthermore, it should be remembered, that tumors of the anaerobic kind can grow without Oxygen-supply anyways, making an O2-rich biological treatment approach even more meaningful, if not a necessity.

Benefits of microecology- testing and enzyme therapy

In a survey of unselected 'walk - in' patients in the mid-eighties, males and females of all ages, without any symptoms or health problems, were chosen to

"The best way to develop cancer is to have a suppressed I weak Immune-System.

The best way to prevent cancer is to build and maintain a strong and healthy Immune-System., participate in a "Cancer-risk screening" test. Approximately 68% of these individuals had clinical-biochemical parameter test results indicating early cancer risks. In an epidemiological approach these 'risk' individuals had a similar history of use of antibiotics during repeat periods of their life and/or also over prolonged periods of time, and with different products – sometimes dating back to their infancy. Further EAV (Electro-Acupuncture -according to- Voll) testing, as introduced Id the U.S. by Dr. Dietmar Schildwaechter prior to 1976, pointed towards the intestinal system as a problem area. In cooperation with researchers and experts in the field of Micro-ecology and in utilizing stool-sample cultures for testing at the Institute for Micro-Ecology at Herborn, Germany, almost without exception abnormal and pathological intestinal flora was diagnosed. When epidemiological surveys revealed the use of cortisone containing products as well, the findings were even more disturbing. Total absence of the important E. coli was found, and pathological 'replacement' flora like Pseudomonas and / or Klebsiella were frequently discovered. This resulted in a paralyzing effect on the all-important lymphatic system that lines the intima of the small and large intestines, ultimately responsible for detoxification of non-organic food additives. Necessary restoration of a normal intestinal flora, requiring Enzymes in sufficient dosages and combined with products recommended by Micro-ecology experts, was possible and could be monitored with the Cancer and Immune Profile blood test. During this important Immune Enhancing normalization of a physiological intestinal flora, the parameter monitoring clearly documented the disappearing cancer risk-numbers accordingly!

"People think that if they simply take vitamins and minerals, they will be healthy, but every vitamin and mineral require an enzyme. You can eat pounds and pounds of vitamins and minerals, but if you don't have the proper enzymes, they won't work. -Lita Lee, Ph. D

Naturally the entire metabolic system of patients improved. » Their Immune Defenses were strengthened: They no longer were susceptible to all kinds of repeat infections like bronchitis, sinusitis, cystitis, and others. Their energy level improved and their outlook on life and health, combined with now a more nutrition-oriented health maintenance type attitude, was usually very noteworthy! It should be mentioned that many patients are buying enzymes over the counter indiscriminately and without guidance or are motivated by television commercials or hear-say from other people. The importance of having the right selection of vitamins in combination with trace minerals, amino acids, and the before mentioned enzymes cannot be overemphasized. An individual -and whenever necessary- adjustable health maintenance program usually costs less than the money spent by many for alcoholic beverages, tobacco products, sweets, or items that are not necessarily beneficial for their health.

Side effects of enzyme intake

It should be mentioned that the intake of plant and animal enzymes, especially in the higher dosage of the GW Formula Proteolytic enzymes is very well tolerated and does not have any side effects. If a patient is originally burdened with a high amount of toxins, due to causes and medications mentioned previously, the initiation of these enzymes at a high dosage may initially lead to symptoms of diarrhea. This is usually a sign of necessary detoxification. Only if a patient is bothered by the initial side effects, the dosage may be reduced, but to resume its normal prescribed dosage after diarrhea subsides. It is of further importance to note that high fluid intake is essential to create the desired detoxification effect. Joseph Issels M.D., one of the widely known German Oncologists used to tell his patients in his first session: "Unless you are able to assure me that you are taking a minimum of 1500 cc or close to 1/2 gallon of fluids per day, I cannot treat you." Should a patient notice symptom like heartburn after enzyme intake, it will usually be an indication of a lack of sufficient fluid intake with these enzymes. Patients will notice and are usually being told ahead-of- time that they will become aware of a certain enzyme smell upon bowel movements as well as upon urination. This is a sign that enzyme intake is beneficially affecting the entire body. Should an individual have difficulty swallowing tablets, they can be crushed and then mixed with something like oatmeal, applesauce , yoghurt, a deliciously blended milk / ice- cream (frozen yoghurt) / and*or fruit shake and this way applied for the patient's benefit The supportive role of enzymes for the effectiveness of vitamins, amino acids and trace minerals taken, is very well known and should be mentioned here again. Without enzyme intake a supplementation that patients do on their own is usually without the desired effect.

Cell-Milieu Medicine

The German physician, Dr. Husso H. Thalman M.D., in Hamburg, Germany, in recent years has given us a better understanding of the effectiveness of metabolic therapies with some of the substances and certainly these enzymes we have addressed in this documentation. He found that the blood serum of a patient may have sufficient trace minerals, trace metals, amino adds, and vitamins, etc. However, in trying to measure the required contents of these live elements in the body's red blood cells, the erythrocytes, he found that they were completely void of these items. His research showed that hair analytical surveys done Tor some years in various places often showed deficiencies or an overload of certain trace elements in the hair samples of patients. In other words, the serum levels, recommending a reduced intake or additional supplementation were strictly based on serum values and did not shed any light on the deficiencies of the body's erythrocyte system. This was caused by a cell membrane which had no permeability and therefore did not allow these enzymes, vitamins, trace minerals and amino acids to reach the body's intermit blood system.

His research, now well documented, published, reported, and presented at medical societies and conventions all over the world proves that not only a supplementation but a supplementation with an increase in the cell wall permeability is necessary' and - possible for a patient to have the benefit of our efforts. His clinical results in patients treated with this new approach and an individualized supplementation program was measured by the CA and Immune Profile blood test and has been interpreted by Dr. Schildwaechter since 1985. The results are stunning and proof of an effective nutritional metabolic and immune enhancing treatment program. If we take into consideration the body's deficiencies and our new ways of making available whatever we supply to organ systems starving in need of regeneration and harmonization.

Pancreatic Enzyme Therapy and Cancer

The history of pancreatic enzyme therapy predates the work in plant enzyme therapy. In 1902, English embryologist John Beard injected pancreatic extracts directly into tumors of cancer patients with therapeutic success. When others tried this method and failed, mainly due to the impurity of the extract preparations, the therapy fell in disrepute. Later in Germany, Dr. Gaschler and Dr. Wolf used enzymes to successfully treat patients with multiple sclerosis, cancer, and viral infections. The two men provided some of the earliest research on enzymes and co-enzymes.

Hector Solorzano del Rio, M.D., D.Sc., Coordinator of the Program for Studies of Alternative Medicine and Professor of Pharmacology of the University of Guadalajara in Mexico, is one of the many physicians who uses pancreatic enzyme therapy. He has treated a wide variety of diseases, inflammatory conditions such as rheumatic disorders, soft tissue trauma, viral infections, arthritis, multiple sclerosis, cancer, and autoimmune diseases, including AIDS. Dosages are given orally on an empty stomach or by injection, and may be combined with plant enzymes.

Dr. Dictmar Schildwaechter M.D.'s specialty in preventing and treating cancer, since 1974, relies heavily on Enzyme Therapy. Pancreatic enzymes, which are produced by mammals, are PROTEASE, AMYLASE and LIPASE. Pancreatic enzymes "function" in the intestines and in the blood. Supplemental pancreatic enzymes can aid digestion in the small and large bowel, sharing the workload of the body's own pancreatic enzymes that are active there. However, for a complete digestive metabolism, the entire chain of enzymes and for all stages of digestion is required.

Our three salivary glands, called Glandula, Glandule Sublingualis and Glandual Parotis, the latter one known for its painful swelling during 'Mumps' are secreting 'sputum' and the first stage of digestion, the moment we put the first bite of food into our mouth. A good chewing-act helps to mix our food with enzymes, already at this early digestive stage, for a complete digestive metabolism with all its stages, the entire chain of special enzymes is required.

The second stage is the enzymatic activity of our stomach juices. They are secreted the moment we swallow, and likewise, ready to receive our chewed and thus "prepared" food for further digestive preparation.

Step three is a most important digestive 'happening': the transfer of predigested food into the next intestinal section. This is called the duodenum. Due to its unusual anatomic shape, the German name for it is: twelve finger gut. Here liver enzymes from the gallbladder and pancreatic enzymes are released and added to step 1 and 2 of pre-digestion, carried on during passage through Jejunum and Ileum (the 'small' intestinal system) as well as through the entire Colon.

It may be of interest to note that the highest concentration of digestive proteolytic and other enzymes in the Duodenum, protects this organ from ever developing primary Cancer. Only metastatic malignancies, growing in from other organs, have been found in the Duodenum by pathologists! Extracting these duodenal enzyme-juices from cadavers and injecting them into lab-animal tumors, had a Cancer-killing effect!

As important as all digestive enzymes are, not only the high volume of pancreatic enzymes, for a normal and beneficial digestion the presence of a healthy intestinal flora is essential. Unfortunately, this sensitive digestive environment is severely damaged in many human beings today due to Mercury-abrasion from Amalgam-fillings, repeat or prolonged use of Antibiotics and toxicity from certain medications. A damaged or pathologic-replacement flora can no longer detoxify and a paralyzed lymphatic system of the intima (inner lining of the intestinal system) 'drains' a patient's immune-system.

Here the need of enzyme supplementation has to assume the important role - and far beyond a digestive aid - of health restoration and immune-enhancement supported by potent remedies containing acidophilus, bifidus and other supplements. Here the medical sub-specialty of Micro-Ecology comes into play.

It has long been recognized; how certain enzyme formulation Gashler-Wolf formula have unusual abilities. They can act as anti-inflammatory-, anti-infectious- and anti-edematous substances. Surgeons have used them pre- and post-surgical with the added benefit of shortening post-surgical recovery of patients. Athletes are using them to reduce the effects of sport-injuries and traumas, as well as for a variety of conditions that handicap certain sport-disciplines.

The FDA (Food and Drug Administration) has recognized the important role of enzymes, but restricted their use as 'dietary supplements' only, according to their labeling as well.

The combination of various enzymes plus other modes of supplementation and care, a healthy diet and avoidance of toxins provides the best preventive as well rehabilitative approach to ailments.

"It cannot be said that a particular enzyme can help a particular illness. Any treatment is multifaceted, requiring various enzymes plus other modes of care, as well as adherence to a healthy diet with adequate raw foods." Howard Loomis, D.C

Conditions Benefited by Proteolytic Enzyme Therapy

Proteolytic enzymes have been shown to be beneficial in a variety of disease conditions, including inflammation, viral disease, multiple sclerosis, and cancer.

Inflammation: Inflammation is a response to noxious stimuli, and is a way the body rids itself of harmful substances. The classical signs of inflammation are pain, redness, swelling, and heat. Once inflammation takes place, however, healing can begin. With sports injuries, enzymes are used to promote inflammation in order to accelerate healing, and taking them before performing athletics can promote faster healing if injury occurs.

Viral Diseases: Viruses have a protein coat, and enzymes are able to initiate reactions that can digest this protective layer so that the viruses can be destroyed. Enzymes also help in the removal of CIC's that are abundant in viral disease. Research also indicates that enzymes are beneficial in the treatment of herpes zoster (shingles), particularly in patients with immune deficiencies. And enzymes can in part counteract the decreased immune function of HIV (human immune deficiency virus) infection.

Multiple Sclerosis: Although the cause of multiple sclerosis is unknown, it has been shown that demyelination, reduction of the fatty covering of the nerves, occurs. Dr. Solorzano tells of a wheelchair - bound patient diagnosed with multiple sclerosis for whom no traditional treatment had helped. Trying proteolytic enzyme therapy, the patient gained strength and could dress himself within one month. After three months, he could work with difficulty, and within six months his symptoms disappeared and he was able to resume a normal, productive life. Similar results were achieved by Dr. Dietmar Schildwaechter., in Jamaica and later in Washington D.C.

Cancer: Proteolytic enzymes can help in the treatment of cancer in several ways: They help to expose a fiber-net on the surface of cancer cells. By destroying this net-structure of fibrin, cancer cells can be recognized as foreign and destroyed by the immune system. Proteolytic enzymes can stimulate natural killer cells, T-cells, and tumor necrosis factor (anticancer agents), all toxic to cancer cells.

By removing the "sticky" net-structure of fibrin found on tumor cells, enzymes reduce the risk of tumors adhering to other areas of the body (i.e., preventing metastasis). And proteolytic enzymes can enter cancer cells in their reproductive phase when they are not completely formed and more susceptible to destruction. Vitamin A increases these effects, as it releases enzymes contained in lysosomes (components of the intercellular digestive system), and is often given in combination with pancreatic enzymes. In Germany and Austria, proteolytic enzyme solutions have been injected directly into tumors, causing them to dissolve.

Pregnancy: During pregnancy most women are not able to take any prescription or over the counter drugs as these may harm the baby and cause damaging side effects. The use of special formula enzymes in a combination with special Vitamin C has no known side effects and may help keep the mother healthy and strong during pregnancy.

The Future of Enzyme Therapy

Future Medicine is an Enzyme-Medicine! There are now over two thousand enzyme therapists in the United States and the field of enzyme therapy is rapidly expanding. "I think enzyme therapy is the wave of the future and will revolutionize the field of nutrition. All preventive therapies will include treatment of enzyme deficiencies and all food supplements will address our need for enzymes," states Dr. Lee.

The use of proteolytic enzyme therapy in the field of medicine has a head start because it already has been the subject of much research in Europe. And Dr. Loomis envisions, "If research funds were currently as available to study all types of enzyme therapy in the United States as they are in Europe, tremendous strides could be taken. The future could be particularly bright for enzyme therapy. Depletion of enzymes leads to a host of chronic diseases that could in part be avoided if we provided the body with the enzymes it needs. As it is, we are not aware of enzyme deficiencies because they take so long to manifest. When there are signs, the body is already in a state of exhaustion. It is here that the future of enzyme therapy lies, in its potentially enormous roll in nutrition and the prevention of chronic degenerative disease."

Where to Find Help

For more guidance as well as information on enzyme therapy & cancer, a specific cancer and immune profile test, as well as European live cell therapy, and the Wolf-Gaschler Formula Enzymes, please contact either:

Specific Cancer and Immune Profile Blood Test

Sovereign Consultants International, Ltd. offers a scientifically calibrated cancer profile and immune spectrum blood test.

This lest is used for die following conditions:

1. To establish a "baseline" of your health and immune status
2. To use as a tool for Prevention of cancer
3. To measure strength or weakness of the immune system and liver
4. To detect early cancer risk
5. To detect exact cancer "happening" in established disease, showing existing primary and/or metastatic cancer activity

6. To monitor response to any treatment chosen

7. To monitor if Remission in cancer patients is achieved

8. To ascertain maintenance of Health and maintenance of Remission

Credits: Thank you to our International expert. Dr. Dietmar Schildwaechter, in sharing his knowledge and experience of over 35 years in preventive and rehabilitative medicine with specialty in cancer, in contributing, in large part the information contained herein. Editing, documentation and select!

Information contributed by Kerstin Schildwaechter, daughter and avid admirer of Dr. Schildwaechter's priceless knowledge. Partial information and layout gathered by Future Medicine Publishing's "Alternative Medicine," by Burton Goldberg Group.

References

Bainbridge, W.S., N.Y. Med. J. 95, 385, 1907

Baird, J., Enzyme Therapy of Cancer, Schatto etc., London, 1911

Blumenthal, F., Z. Krebsforsch. 10, 137, 1910 Campbell, I. T., J. Amer., med. Ass. p. 1030, 1907 Christiani, A. von, Z. Krebsforsch. 47,176, 1939; Enzymologica 28, 163, 1965;

Enzymologica 28, 235, 1965;

Enzymologica 29, 11, 1965;

Enzymologica 34, 162, 1968

Cleaves, H.M., Med. Rec. 70, 91, 1906 Curtefield, A., Brit. Med. J., Oct. 1907

Duprey, H., New Orleans Med. a, Surg. J. July 1907 Freund, E. Wein. med. Wschr. 12, 1934

Freund, E. Wein. klin. Wschr. 46, 1576, 1933

Gaschler, A., Parenterale Fermenttherapie maligner Tumoren, Ulm, Haug Verlag, 1961 Goeth, R.A., J. Amer. Med. Ass. 1907

Hald. P.T., Lancet II, 1371, 1907

Kretz, J„ Wein. klin. Wschr. 6, 1936

Little, W. L. A., J. Amer. Med. Ass. page 1724, 1908 Marsden, A., Gen. Prac. 22, 1908

Physick, A., etc., Pharmacotherapeutics, D.A. Appleton, N.Y. 1928 Pusey, W.A., J. Amer. Med, Ass. 46,1763, 1906

Shaw-McKenzie, J., Brit. Med. J. 1,715, 1906 Sagiroglu, N., Amer. J. Obstetr. a. Gyn. 85, 454, 1963

This chapter is excerpted from Enzyme Therapy by Max Wolf, M.D.

Basic Notions in Microscopy

by Gaston Naessens

For a long time now, the microscope has been an invaluable tool of precision in research laboratories and in the general industries altogether. The classical microscope uses visible light. Research for substituting that kind of radiation has been attempted and from that grew the ultra-violet, the infra-red and more recently the electronic microscopy.

As early as the 19th century, polarized light was used in microscopy. Maybe in the near future will protonic microscopy conquer this area of research. Recently there has been research directed at bringing in different optical phenomena to the service of microscopy: interference, phasing contrast, etc.

These possibilities are seriously being studied and we can expect that in the next few years we will witness new developments in that area of work. The basic principle behind the microscope is that it makes possible the observation of objects that are otherwise too small to be observed by the naked eye.

The dimension of the smallest object that we can see with the naked eye is limited by the acuteness of our eyesight. The capacity of the eye under normal conditions is in range of 1° angle. (That is when the lighting is normal, the eye not tired and at a good distance from this point of focus.)

For example, two parallel lines will be seen as separated when the angle for which our eye is the summit (and both sides apply) to an angle superior to 1°. Conventionally, a middle- age observer with normal eyesight must place the object at a distance which we call minimum distinct vision distance which is a distance of 25 centimeters.

The separating power in that case would be 75 microns. A magnifying glass will allow us to improve the separating power by diminishing the minimum distance of observation of the object, and it will do so by increasing the width of the angle that we are now observing. But this improvement will not allow us to reach higher magnifications.

Indeed, it is necessary that the outer pupil of the instrument be sufficiently far from the face of exit of the optical system so that it may coincide with the entrance pupil of the observer's eye. As soon as a simple magnifying glass reaches a magnification of 20X, that becomes possible.

The difference is that a microscope helps out the pupil with a composed system, (outside of a complicated optical system) and actually allows a reach of 0.02 microns under visible light. With these methods, if we use electrons instead of protons, which forms the elementary particles of light, this limit is pushed back to a few angstroms (10/1000 micron).

Measures of length

m dm mm   M   mp   A
cm

	10	1 00	1	0
		00	0	0
1000		00	0	0
	66		0	0

1 millimicron

1 anameter

1 micron

1 millimeter

1 Angstrom Cosmic rays

= 10 Angstroms

= 1 millimicron

= 1,000 millimicron

= 10,000 Angstroms

= 1,000 microns

= 1,000,000 millimicron

= 10,000,000 Angstroms

= 1/10,000,000 millimeter

= 0.0002 Angstroms or 2/10,000 Angstroms

When we use photons, this limit is pushed back to an even smaller fraction of an angstrom. The microscope is therefore considered to be an instrument which gives us the image of an object by simply magnifying its intimate structure.

There exists other methods of observing the intimate structure of an object. Those methods, being indirect ones, require the study of diffraction phenomena produced by the object. The microscope is then used in an indirect manner. Light (as it is the case for all types of radiations that allow viewing of an image) is separated in two parts; the corpuscular and the undulatory aspects.

To create an image, we can use all radiations offering an undulatory aspect. These radiations are named infra-red light, visible light, ultra-violet light, electrons and protons. In fact, only the ones just mentioned have been used, although others, X-Rays and Gamma Rays belong to the same category of radiations.

The difference between photonic microscopy (achieved through the undulatory aspect of light), and corpuscular microscopy (electronic microscopy), is less obvious than what was first believed. It is due to the fact that in a range of various phenomena it is at times the corpuscular aspect which is most dominant and at other times it is the undulatory aspect.

In looking back at these basic principles, it appears that the resolution (linear separating power) depends on the angle (numerical opening) as well as on the wavelength of light. We have thus directed our research to find out what the limit of the resolution power could be. In other words, what is the extreme limit beyond which it becomes impossible to perceive the distance between the two lines?

Let's take the simplest example possible, that of two parallel streaks. We can add up the value of the sinus of the angle formed by the diffracted beams and the direct beam.

The value is equal to the relation between wavelength of the light ray and the distance between the streaks. Therefore, for each specific wavelength, it is possible to find the different values of the angle for each distance separating the streaks.

We now know that there are two ways of pushing back the limits of resolution; first the numerical opening, second the wavelength of the light ray. The optical industry, with its advanced technology comes out regularly with new findings in the field of numerical openings. We therefore directed our research more toward the second parameter of the subject: the wavelength of the light ray.

THE NAESSENS SOMATOSCOPE

In order to obtain a higher resolution we have invented an instrument with the underlying principle residing in an increase of the frequency of light. Two light sources, one incandescent with a wavelength of 3,300 angstroms, the other ultra-violet of 1,850 angstroms start pulsating, producing a third wavelength. This wave goes through a monochromator which produces a ray. This ray is exposed to a magnetic field, the Zeemann effect, which splits it into parallel rays.

One of these rays is treated by a Kerr cell which increases its frequency. This cell is then stimulated by a step generator-oscillator at frequencies which vary from 250 to 1,200 megahertz.

The modulation of a visible light at frequencies ranging from 250 to 1,200 megahertz produces a basic frequency ranging from 250 to 1,200 megahertz, but also harmonics at higher frequencies (if we use light in the order of 2,000 A).

The resulting beam has particular characteristics in terms of general behavior and penetrating action. It is this source of light, invisible to the naked eye, that analyzes the image.

Although the technical considerations are not to be a part of this presentation, we are nevertheless allowed to say that the resolution of this instrument is in the order of 150 A and the power of its magnification varies from 2,000 to 30,000 X.

The image observed is produced by rays that are diffracted from the different diopters forming the object. The structures thus appear in light colors on a black background. Despite the more frequent use of new methods of investigation in the world of microscopy it is obvious that this new concept is of the utmost choice.

This method proves itself to be very superior to any other when it comes to studying uncolored and extremely reduced structures which are on the limit or inferior to the normal separating power of a photonic microscope.

The possible identification of micro-organisms in the blood, in the secretions or in the homogenized tissues could largely widen the horizons of medicine.

THE DISCOVERY OF THE SOMATIC

As you know the electron microscope allows the observation of fixed tissues (or dead tissues) whereas the somatoscope lets us observe live substances.

That is how I have been able to observe ultramicroscopic organisms in the blood smaller than viruses, (organisms that haven't yet been observed by most scientists). These organisms that I have named "somatids" have very specific characteristics such as their charge, their density and their immortality. Furthermore, they pass on the genetic characters of the species.

I can watch them live and develop as their forms and appearances change. They move without ever agglomerating or piling up because they bear an electric charge.

Their nucleus is positive and their membrane is negative so that when two somatids come close to one another there is an automatic repulsion in the same manner as when you try to put together the negative poles of two magnets.

I have also observed that health is directly related to the evolution of the cycle of the somatid. The discovery of the somatid is a major one concerning life as much for the vegetable kingdom as for the animal kingdom.

THE NAESSENS ULTRAMICROSCOPE

We now understand that the image obtained through ultramicroscopy is the result of diffraction phenomena that are created by the undulatory movement of the light rays as they hit the objects that are not capable of emitting light by themselves.

Abbe's theory advances that a basic distinction is established between the image of the objects that are self-light-producing and the ones that are not. The self-light-producing objects consist of points which in themselves constitute independent moving centers.

So it is that only the rays leaving from a same point produce amongst themselves interference phenomena. To the contrary, the light waves that leave from each of the points forming the object are somehow inconsistent with each other and their basic waves cannot interfere with one another.

The image of a point of light that will be seen through a lens will be made of a bright central point surrounded by diffraction circles with a rapidly decreasing light intensity. The size of those circles will depend upon the angle of aperture of the lens and the diameter of the diaphragm.

If we are talking about an object instead of a dot, each dot diffracted from this object will give an image surrounded with excessively small diffraction circles. We know that the light rays emitted by each point are independent and cannot interfere with each other.

Therefore, every picture for each point is formed independently without allowing the elementary images to influence one another and create interference and diffraction phenomena.

About the non-self-light-producing objects; to be able to obtain an image, those objects must be lit with a light source, but they work through absorption, refraction and diffraction on the rays that are supplied by the said light source.

Here the conditions for the creation of an image are totally different. Each point forming the object is created by the convergence of the rays arriving from all points of the light source used on the object. Those rays are independent from one another and by opposition to the ones mentioned earlier, they cannot give a diffracted picture of the dots of the object.

To the contrary, the rays coming from the different points of the object can interfere with each other. The object acts as a diffraction network on the rays arriving from the light source and first gives a diffracted image of the source.

From this last image rays are emitted and their interference produces an image of the object. This image is therefore a secondary phenomenon, subordinate to the production of the diffraction image. Thus, came the name that was given to it by Abbe: secondary image.

Starting from this theory, we have put together a condenser that resembles the cardioid condenser used by many optical device makers except that our condenser gives a much more oblique effect, then allows us to obtain a diffraction image.

Because the diffraction image penetrates more completely into the lens, this secondary image is much more detailed. We can say that the resolution power depends first and foremost on the angle of aperture of the lens. The bigger the angle, the bigger will be the portion of the diffraction image that will penetrate the microscope.

Up until today, the ultra-microscope has been of very little use to the biological sciences, at least from a practical point of view. The main reason for it being that it is impossible to determine the form of the object that is being observed.

This serious inconvenience is now eliminated with the arrival of this considerable improvement. Furthermore, the main advantage of this system is its simplicity.

Up until now the somatoscope was a unique model. After being criticized about it I decided to start working on the distribution of a condenser that would allow everyone to observe the somatidian cycle. That condenser is now available to everyone.

With this condenser it is possible to obtain ultramicroscopic vision even with a light source as weak as 20 watts. It is of course obvious that the more intense the light, the better the vision will be.

We can't speak here of an increase in the resolution, but rather of an ultramicroscopic vision beyond the microscope's normal resolution allowing for the observation of somatids.

This condenser is made of many mobile elements that can be adapted to all brands of microscopes. The best observations can be obtained with, a 100X immersion lens and eyepieces of 15X or more. A device to increase the magnification by 1.5X will allow for magnification in the order of 21500X. Furthermore, adapting a videotape machine to it represents no difficulty.

The condenser consists first of a central body with sliding lens-holder which allows us to adjust the height of the lens for all microscopes.

When the right height has been achieved, we tighten the ring in order for it to stay in place. We have adapters for all makes of microscopes.

This discovery will help bring into light the different stages of the somatidian cycle. That will open the door to true disease prevention, by helping us detect the terrains that are predisposed to disease.

CONCLUSION

What comes out of all our discussion is that the knowledge related to the somatid and its cycle has allowed us to establish the relationship that exists between the forms that have been observed under the somatoscope and the degenerative diseases. These many observations have rendered it possible to propose a very promising adjuvant therapy.

Furthermore, the condenser that was presented to you gives access to the somatidian theory and its applications for all scientists and therapists who wish to contribute to the well- being of humanity.

THE PHYSIOLOGY OF BLOOD AS A TISSUE

A Review of Research by

Le Centre Experimental de Recherches Biologiques de I'Estrie Inc. 1

by John W. Mattingly 2

At a Symposium titled, "Controversial Aspects of AIDS" held at Hunter College, December 6, 1986, Francoise Naessens presented recent findings by the Centre Experimental de Recherches Biologiques de L'Estrie, Inc. (C.E.R.B.E.) in their preliminary research with individuals having AIDS, Kaposi's sarcoma or a combination of these two diseases.

Since the works of C.E.R.B.E. are not widely known, the editor has elected to incorporate Francoise Naessens' presentation with a review of prior research by this unique laboratory.

John W. Mattingly, August 17, 1987

During the past 20 years the Centre Experimental de Recherches Biologiques de I'Estrie, Inc (C.E.R.B.E.) has extensively investigated the physiology of mammalian blood.

Their research policy might well be called dialectic, in the sense that emphasis has been placed on direct observation of living processes, with maximal attention to learning from the form and function of the subject under conditions of minimal intervention. Their position reflects the scientific philosophy of Claude Bernard, Alexis Carrel and Hans Selye.

C.E.R.B.E.'s research policy evolved out of perfection of an extraordinary light microscope in the early 1960's. Using a combination of ultraviolet innovation and the dark-field condenser, it was possible to observe certain classes of living specimens at magnifications as high as 30,000X.

More important, resolution of the order of 150 angstroms was realized. The high magnifications proved difficult to utilize on a routine basis. Given high resolution, magnifications of 3000X to 4500X have been adequate for defining physical details and physiological processes of the utmost importance.

Supplementary instrumentation for the higher magnifications was destroyed by accident several years ago. It has not been replicated due to the pressure of more urgent work and limited resources.

The C.E.R.B.E. microscope was perfected more than 30 years prior to recent findings that the assumed limitations of magnification and resolution of light microscopies are simply not true.

Its singular, unique design is based on a fundamental principle with which few modern- day microbiologists are familiar, the dark-field condenser. To grasp the significance of the microbiological paradigm established by C.E.R.B.E., it is of far greater importance to understand certain historical facts about dark-field microscopy than it is to debate just how such high magnifications and resolution can be had with a light microscope.

The dark-field condenser was invented in 1837 by a Reverend J. B. Reade. With this lens system certain details can be seen in living specimens which cannot be seen clearly with other systems. However, it is not well suited for examining stained specimens, a major deterrent to its popularity.

Few researchers have been disposed to base their works on an unconventional instrument and the relatively limited body of knowledge accumulated with the dark-field microscope remains foreign to the contemporary microbiologist.

C.E.R.B.E.'s dedication to research based on their unique combination of ultraviolet technology and the dark field condenser has revitalized an old methodology and created a new perspective of living matter.

So much can be seen with this instrument that conventional fixing, staining, labeling and tracing practices have been viewed by C.E.R.B.E. as counterproductive for establishing a new paradigm in microbiology.

Excessively invasive, if not destructive, these widely used techniques, devised to extend the range of information available with conventional light microscopes, obliterate crucial details and processes of living specimens.

Conventional fixing and staining are rarely practiced at C.E.R.B.E. Colors seen in original prints of photomicrographs to follow have been produced by manipulations of the microscope lighting system.

The absence of familiar laboratory techniques, together with the unconventional microscope lighting system employed by C.E.R.B.E., have made it extremely difficult for contemporary microbiologists to perceive that this body of research might disclose invaluable new perspectives and ask a crucial new class of questions deserving careful exploration.

It represents an entirely different biological paradigm which can perhaps be understood only on its own terms.

THE SOMATID

The works of Antoine Bechamp [3], one of the earliest of the rare devotees of dark-field microscopy, are reflected by the findings of C.E.R.B.E. With the dark-field condenser, Bechamp found tiny bright motile bodies in the circulatory fluids of all of the many evolved life forms he examined.

Early in his adventures in biology, Gaston Naessens, C.E.R.B.E.'s principal researcher, was attracted to dark-field microscopy. Upon seeing the same entity Bechamp had seen scores of years before, he was driven to improve the microscopes at his disposal to better define its properties. Satisfying himself that it had physiologic functions in the blood of mammals, he named it "somatid," being unaware of Bechamp's works at the time.

Confirming the presence of the somatid in the blood of all healthy humans, C.E.R.B.E. postulates that in conditions of health a modulated necessary quantity of somatids originate in the erythrocytes, the various kinds of white cells, the thymus and other formative organs such as the lymph system.

In conditions of disease an additional self-perpetuating mode of somatid production becomes established to the detriment of the host organism. This will be elaborated upon in the following discussion of culturing. Varying in size between 50 and 150 angstroms, the larger of these cells are clearly visible in properly prepared fresh blood specimens with ordinary research- grade dark-field, light-field or phase contrast microscopes.

In dark-field they appear as motile, refractive bodies, their motion not being Brownian. They do not fit the description of virus, viroid's, prions or any of the 250-odd "bodies" listed in Dorland's Illustrated Medical Dictionary.

It is anticipated that further research will show that not only do somatids occur in a range of sizes, but that their properties or functions vary depending on their origin.

The somatid has been viewed by C.E.R.B.E. as an autonomous entity. Bechamp postulated his "microzymas" was an anatomical element. It might also be termed a physiologic component of the blood.

Others have perceived of this micro-body as a symbiont, a useful view in light of recent attention given to the phenomenon of symbiosis, most notably by Lynn Margulis[4] at Boston University.

One medical researcher has called the entity an "obligate symbiont," one whose true properties cannot be studied when isolated from its symbiotic relationship.

Weighing the idea of obligate symbiont, the question arises as to why this particle does not qualify as an anatomical element of the same category as red and white cells, as postulated by Bechamp.

The question is partially answered by the fact that C.E.R.B.E. and others have demonstrated this mysterious entity has bacteria-like properties under certain conditions of disease.

Prevailing views in physiology, bacteriology and hematology cannot encompass the idea of a bacterium as a symbiont in the blood stream, though in fact this may be the truth of the matter.

CULTURING

Only with difficulty can useful quantities of free somatids be isolated directly from whole blood samples. C.E.R.B.E. has found a means for extracting quantities of an extraordinary cell from whole blood which they have named "telocyte."

It has been demonstrated that the telocyte will culture and that it can be broken down into component cells which also culture. The component cells exhibit the same general characteristics of somatids.

Instructions for the extraction technique were made available by the laboratory in 1970 in a house paper titled Immunology. Beginning with 7 ml of fresh whole blood, plasma is eliminated by centrifuge, the red cells are hemolyzed and following a sequence of rinses, final centrifuging produces a small (less than 3 mm diameter) nearly black precipitate of teiocytes.

In a temporary medium of distilled water, the telocyte appears in the dark-field as a circular bright uniformly granular cell 3 to 8 microns in diameter. The larger cells approximate the size of RBCs and the smaller ones the size of poly-nuclear nuclei. Some exhibit motile granulations.

C.E.R.B.E.'s extraction procedure appears specifically suited for isolating a cell of extraordinary high strength and density. The telocyte is not found as an independent entity in fresh blood specimens.

It is postulated to be the nucleus of one of the known kinds of white cells, the nucleus possibly undergoing morphological change during the extraction process. The integrity of known white cells is destroyed by the extraction process.

The telocyte may be cultured in a suitable medium, its growth being characterized by the same stages of evolution as will be described below for the somatid. The telocyte does not become active in culture for three or four weeks, whereas the somatid component shows growth within one week.

It has been shown that the telocyte can be broken down into elements which have the same appearance and motility as the characteristic somatid cell seen in fresh blood specimens. Breaking up the relatively large dense telocyte cells requires positive grinding pressures with a homogenizer against the cells in the bottom of the test tube.

Somatids are obtained by breaking down telocyte cells culture in a suitable medium. They propagate a variety of forms in sequences dependent on properties of the medium. A growth hormone is created in the culture which has been classed by C.E.R.B.E. as a "trephone" after the usage of Alexis Carrel, physiologist and surgeon (1873-1944) 5.

That a hormone should be produced by a somatid culture is not extraordinary. It has been found recently that soil bacteria produce quantities of plant-growth hormones in the rhizosphere ® and abscisic acid, a hormone produced by plants, has been identified in rat and pig brains.

It is postulated by C.E.R.B.E. that in a rich anaerobic medium the culture can contain many if not all of the forms shown diagrammatically in Figure 1 which depicts a complex reproductive cycle incorporating a combination of a number of processes associated with acknowledged pleomorphic bacterial species.

It is further postulated that stages 1 through 3 of this cycle occur naturally within the human circulatory system in conditions of health and that in conditions of disease there is an absence of essential inhibitors and the complete cycle becomes established.

Figure 1,

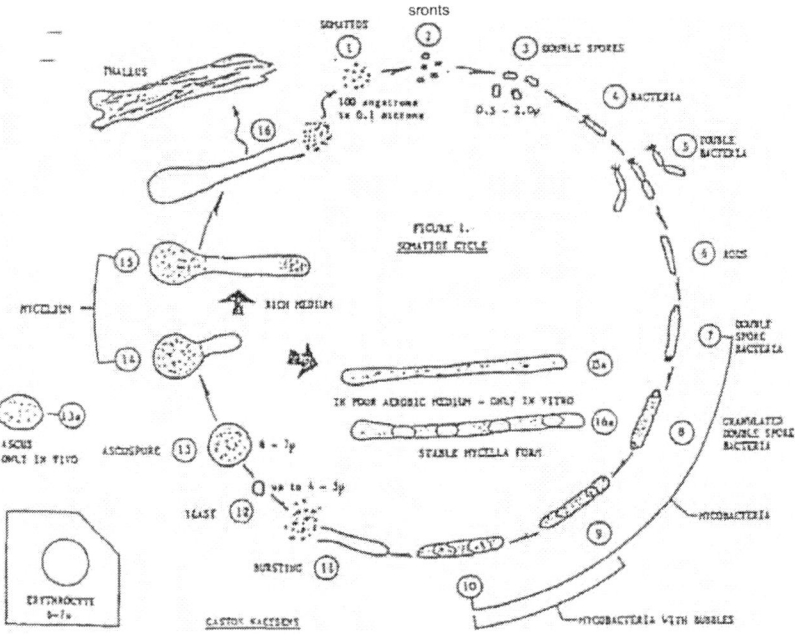

Photograph 1. A somatic! culture at 3,000X. Many forms in the culture have been captured in detail at higher magnification. Calling this a "somatic! culture " means the culture begins with somatids and additional numbers of this entity are produced by the complex cycle.

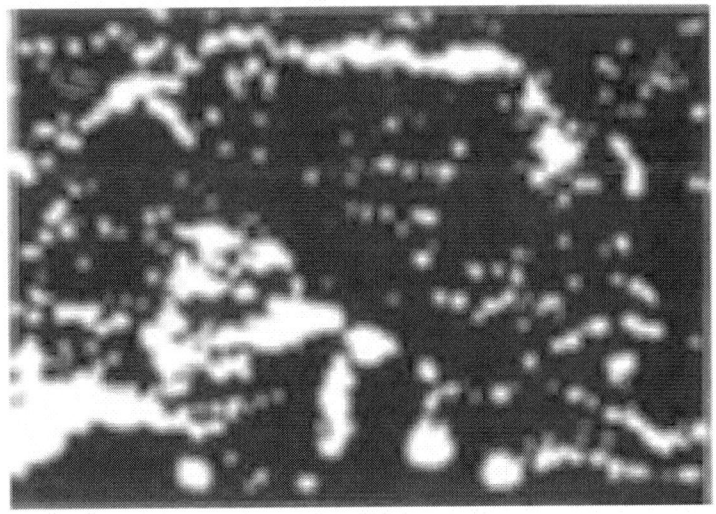

Photograph 2. The somatid culture at 20.000X (stage 1). The largest cells at the top are spores. The larger of the bright cells across the center are large somatids. (Stages 1 and 2).

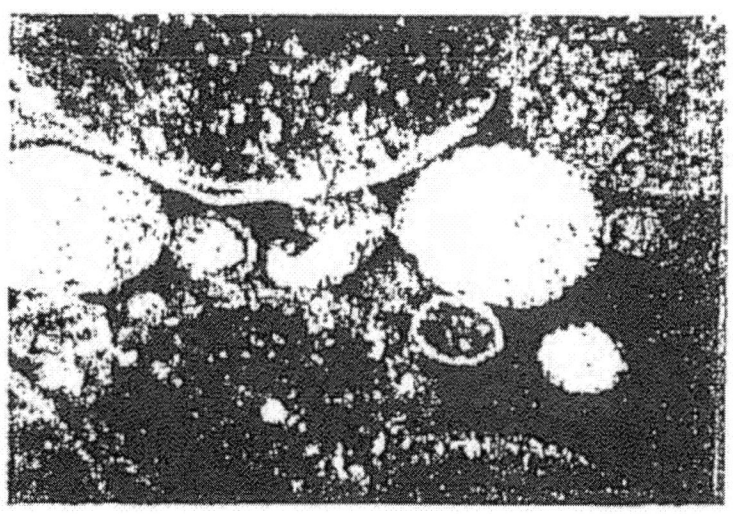

Photograph 3. A large spore (stage 2), 30.000X.

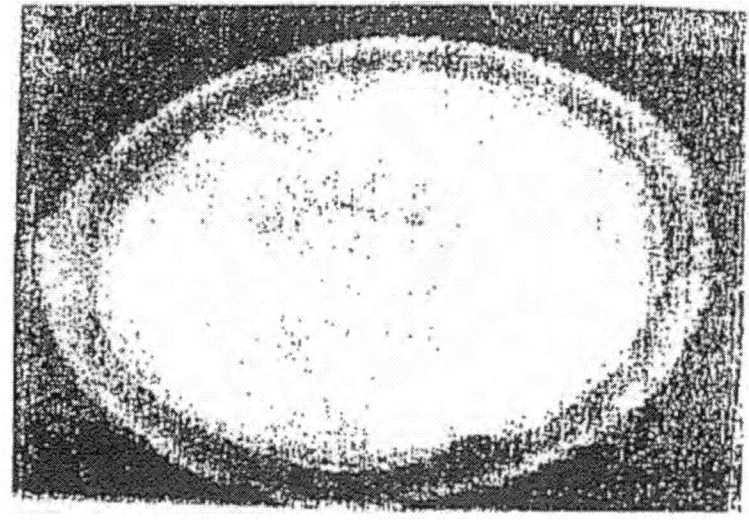

Photograph 4. Double spore (stage 3). 30.000X.

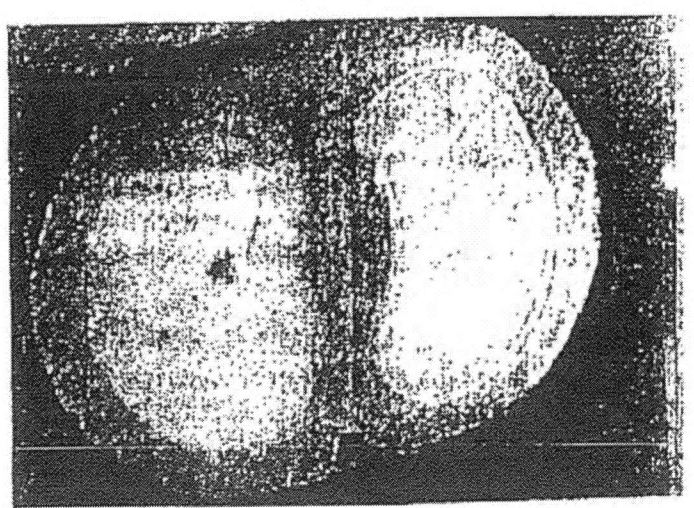

Photograph 5. Spore in the process of dividing. 30,000X.

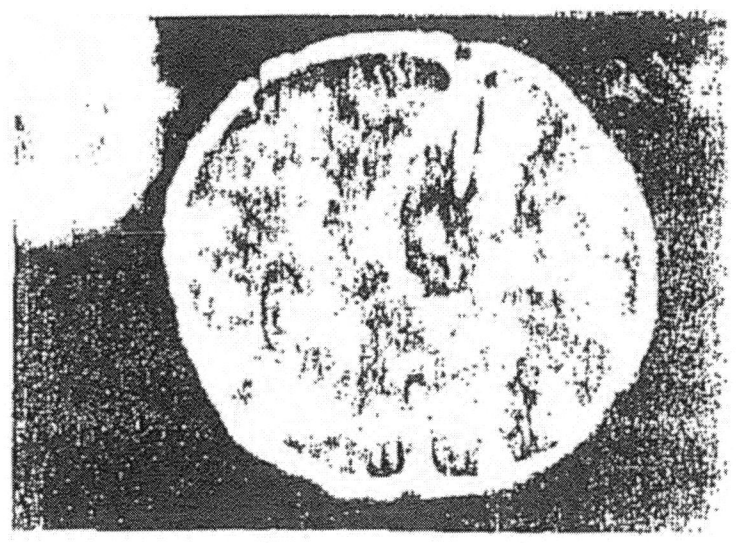

Photograph 6. The cell on the left is a spore in the process of dividing and in the two on the right the internal division is complete. 25,000X.

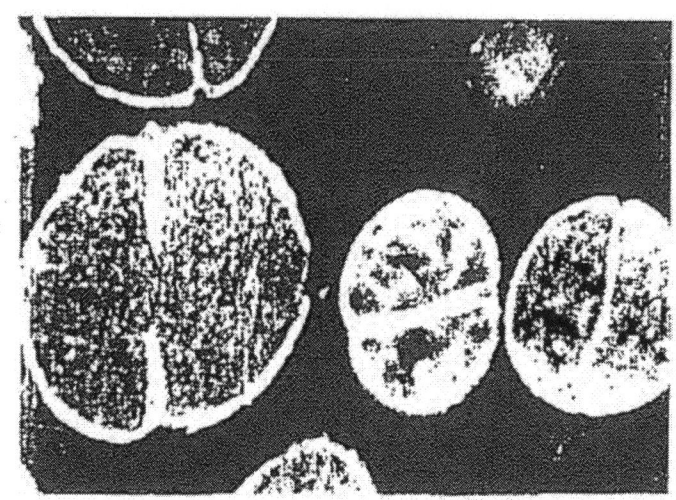

Photograph 7. The mycobacteria with inclusions. 16,000X. (Stages 7-10)

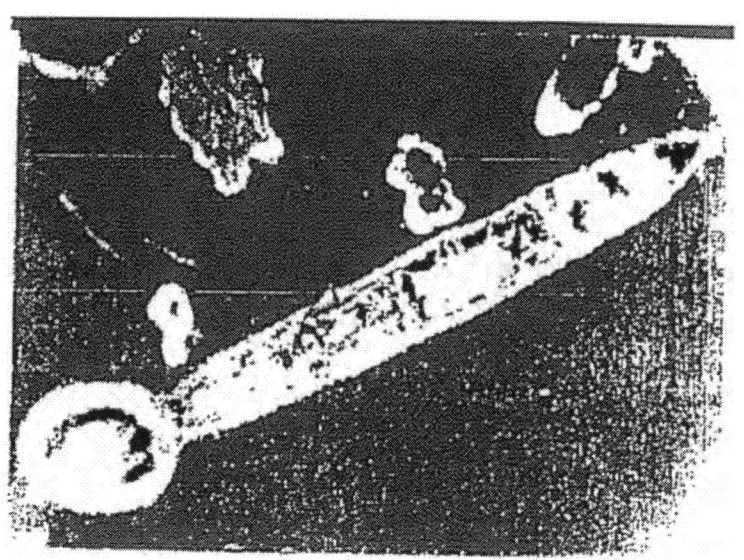

Photographs. Two ascospores. 23,000X. (Stage 13)

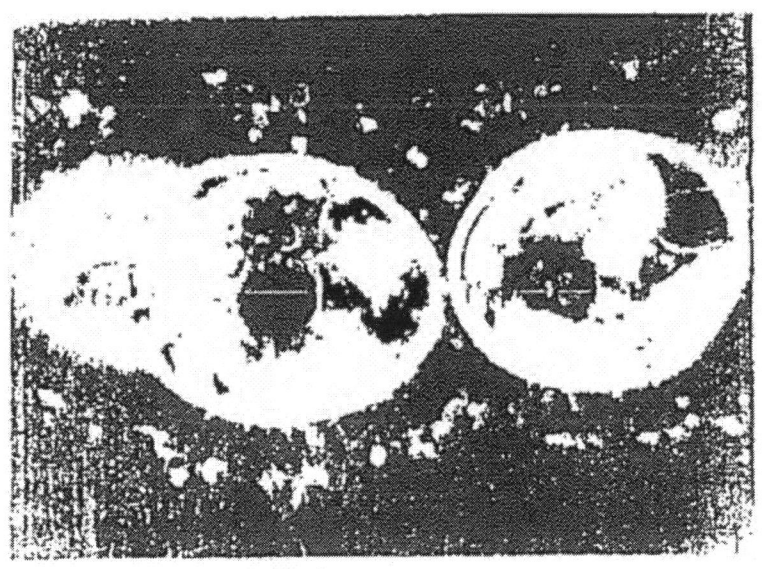

Photograph 9. (20,000X). An ascospore which has evolved from the yeast form in stage 12 and will begin to form a thallus (stage 14) as shown in photo 10, or evolve into a stable mycelia form (stage 15a and 16a) as shown in photo 14, depending on the culture medium. 20,000X.

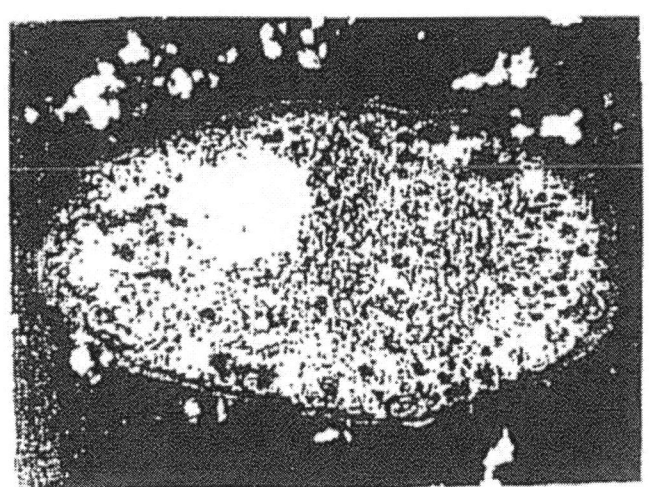

Photograph 10. In the center is a striking view of an ascus with a well-developed thallus (stage15) which has not yet become filled with cytoplasm from the body of the ascus. 3,000X. This is clearly a classical mycelium form which will evolve and burst.

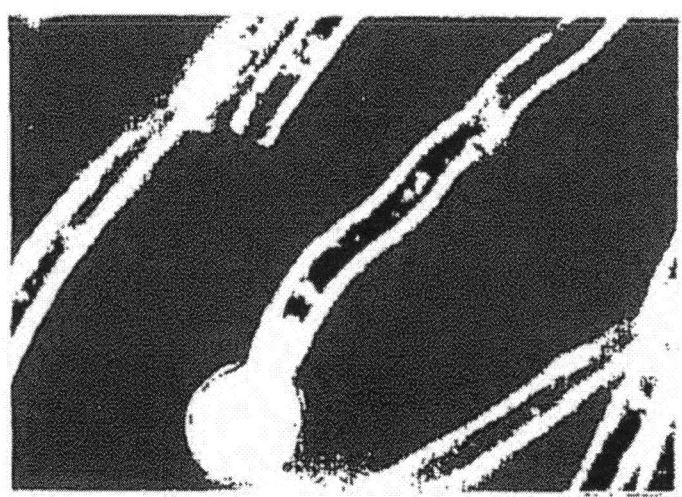

Photograph 11. The ascus has continued the production of cytoplasm and expelled it into the thallus by peristaltic action. The thallus is now full and the ascus (on the right) has collapsed. 3,000X. The dark area between the filled thallus and the spent ascus is the peristaltic valve mechanism which can be seen clearly in photo 56 at 30,000X.

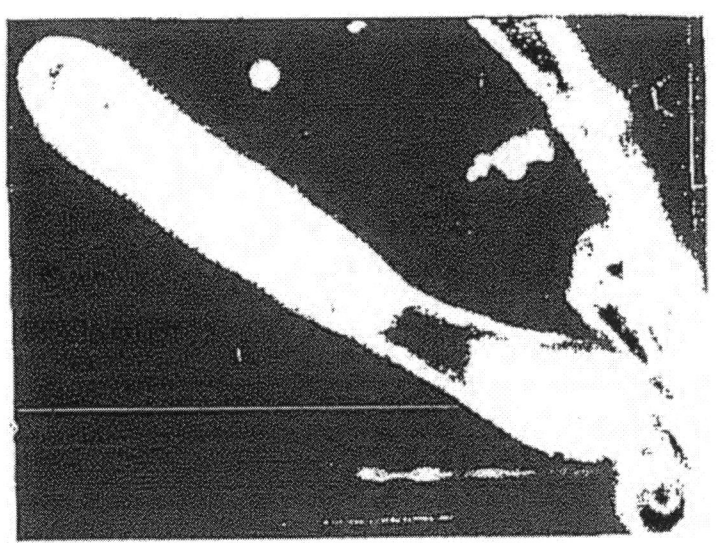

Photograph 12. Explosion at the tip of the filled thallus releasing a large quantity of new primary somatids into the medium. This source of additional quantities of somatids stimulates the quantitative activity of the full 16-stage cycle. It is postulated that trephone production is thereby increased and that an excess of this growth hormone causes the normal rate of body cell division to slip out of control, leading to entrenchment of the condition known as cancer.

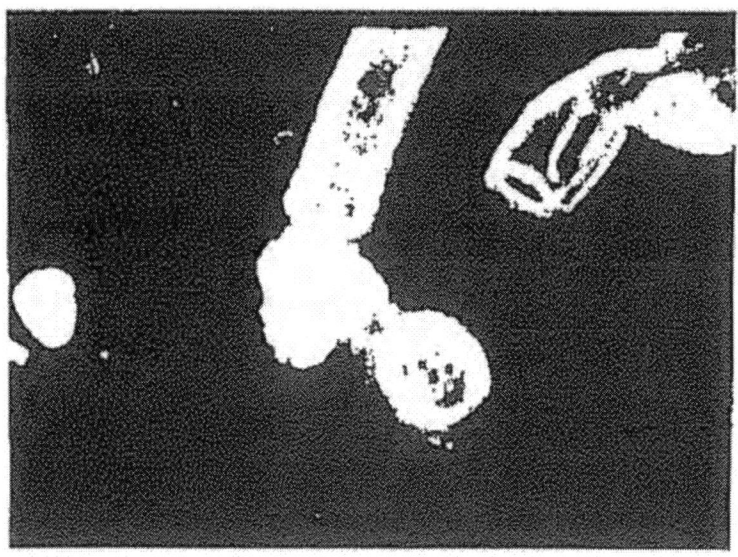

Photograph 13. The spent thallus, a lifeless mycelial waste product often seen by hematologists and called a staining "artifact."

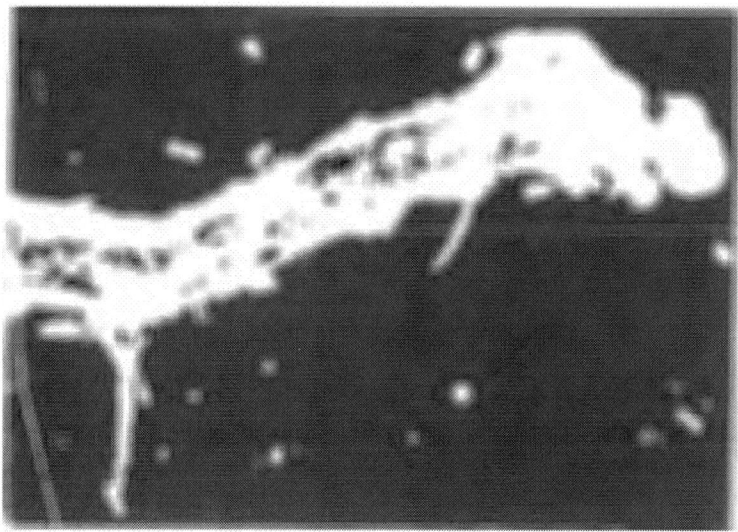

Photograph 14. In a deficient aerobic culture, the ascospore at stage 14 reverts to a stable mycelia form. 6,500X.

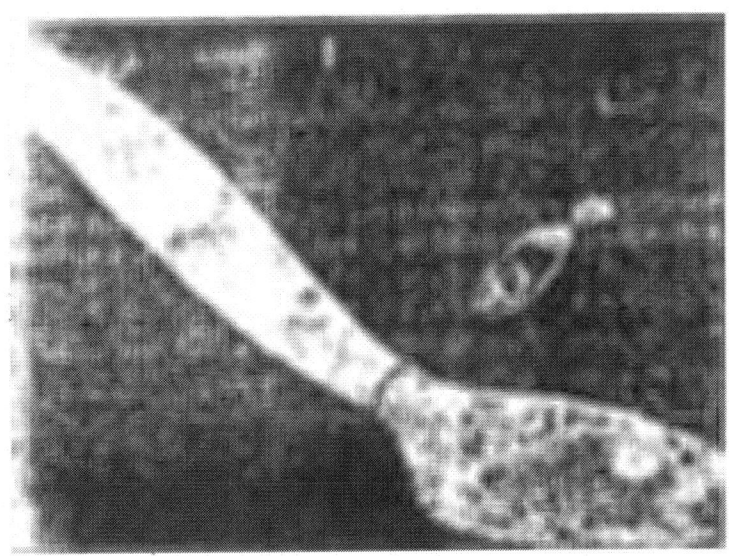

Photograph 15. Details of a portion to the left of center of the stable mycelia. 30,000X, Dormant cultures of this nature have been reactivated after being held at variable ambient temperatures for more than 20 years and after deep-freezing, autoclaving and exposure to intense radiation.

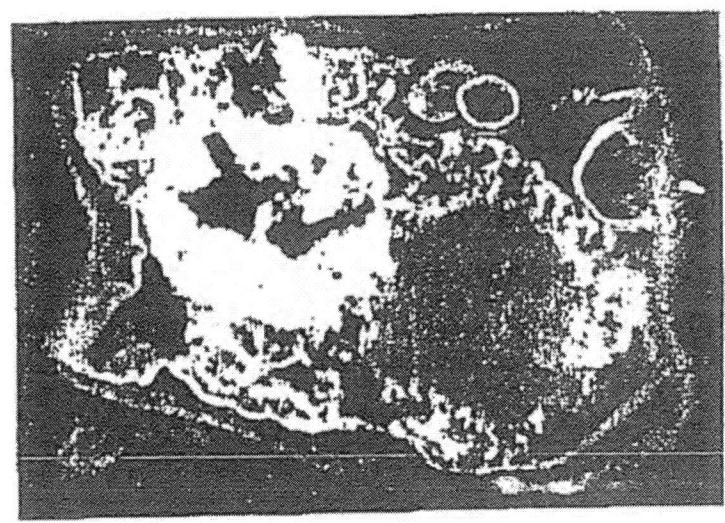

Photograph 16. The resistant spore form in which these cultures survive. 23,000X.

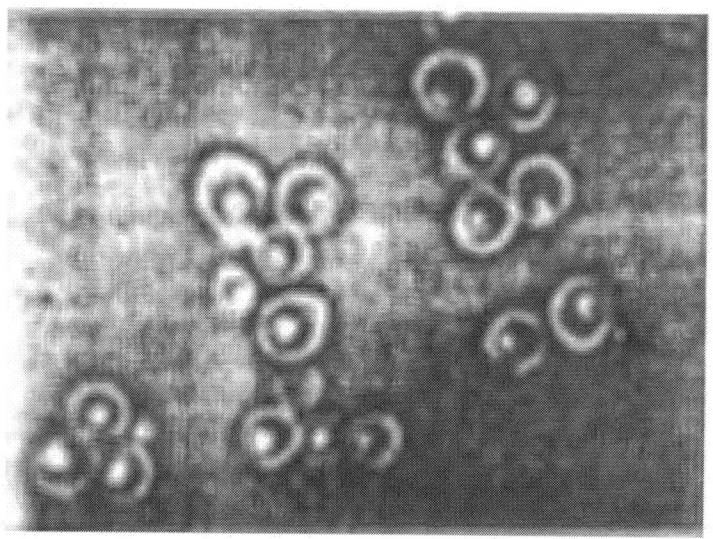

Photograph 17. The same culture at 23,000X.

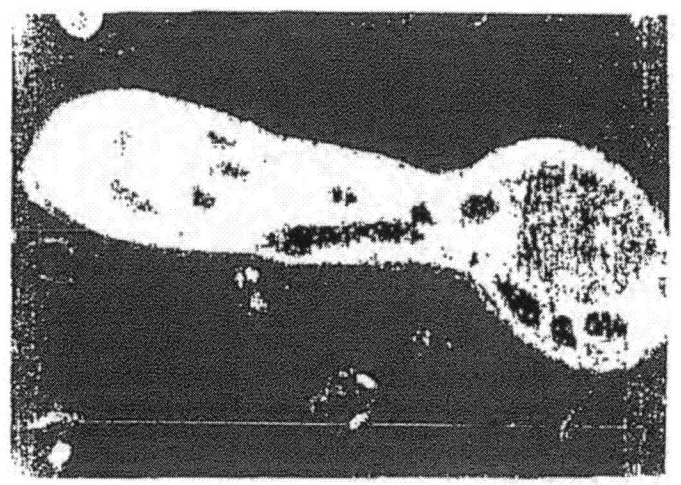

IMMUNOLOGICAL PROPERTIES

Preliminary studies by C.E.R.B.E. show that somatids obtained from the telocyte cell have immunological properties. When injected into the vein of 8 to 10-pound rabbits at the rate of 4.0×10^6 cells daily for 10 days there is no anaphylactic reaction.

Erythropoiesis and polychromatophylla are stimulated. Following 10 days of injections, certain genetic characteristics, such as color of hair, are modified if the donor Is of a different species.

If cross-injections are made between a white rabbit and a black rabbit of different strains their immune systems become matched to a degree allowing each to accept a successful skin graft from the other without the use of immunosuppressive drugs.

Immunity is the so-called system by which the individual organism sustains integrity in constant interaction with the total environment. Few immune systems are born totally equal and in the final analysis the phenomenon remains a mystery to medical science.

Much Is known about how to suppress (kill) immunity for organ transplants, while relatively little is known about how to make the system work better. C.E.R.B.E.'s experiments showing that a culturable entity isolated from the blood has the property of conveying immunological and/or genetic specificity from one organism to another holds a potential for enormous advances in the biological sciences.

WHOLE BLOOD STUDIES

Research by C.E.R.B.E has disclosed a connection between the somatid and the morphology of erythrocytes. Slide preparation for this kind of observation differs from the smear technique commonly used in hematology.

A small quantity of blood Is taken directly from a punctured fingertip with the center of a slide. Immediately, a cover slip is gently lowered on the specimen and examination Is made during the following ten minutes. Held to the light, the slide has a pale orange color.

On slides prepared from healthy subjects an obvious but small number of bright mobile somatids are always visible in the dark background among optically void RBCs.

If a larger specimen is drawn from a healthy subject, washed and placed in hypotonic saline and a slide prepared and examined Immediately as described above, somatids will not be found in the saline medium.

Those normally present have been removed by washing. Soon, both motile and non- motile inclusions begin to appear within the previously optically empty RBCs and a few free somatids are seen.

Crenation follows, bacterial forms evolve within the RBCs and escape through the membrane, frequently appearing as chains or rod-like flagella before breaking free of the RBC membrane.

Within a period of thirty minutes, at ambient temperatures, an enormous number of somatids appear in the background together with a variety of bacterial forms. In whole, unwashed blood specimens, if the microscope stage is heated to 46° C, this sequence of events occurs within 15-20 minutes. Without the stage heater, from one to four hours of patient observation of whole blood specimens is required, depending on ambient temperatures.

Micrographs 18 through 24 show details of some of the events described above as seen in whole unwashed blood specimens.

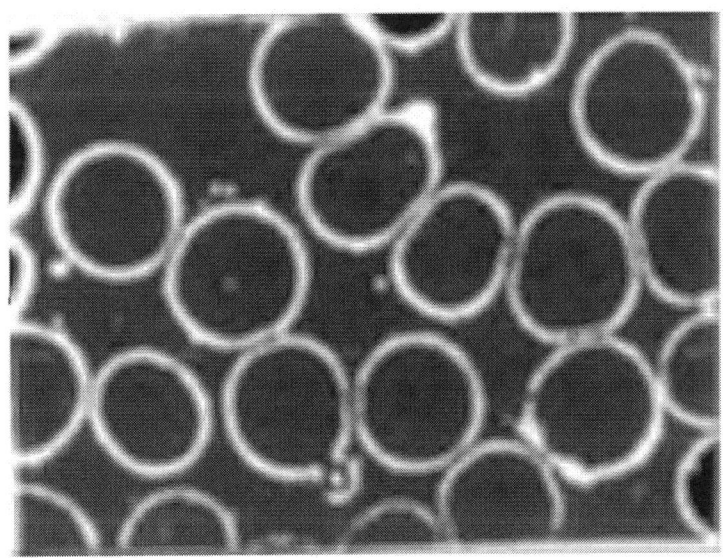

Photograph 18. Below and just to the left of center is a RBC forming a bud with a centrosome. Just above center is another cell beginning to bud. The small bright bodies in the background are somatids. 4,500X.

Photograph 19. A more advanced stage of budding. The centrosome is well developed. In the background are somatids and spores. 4,500X.

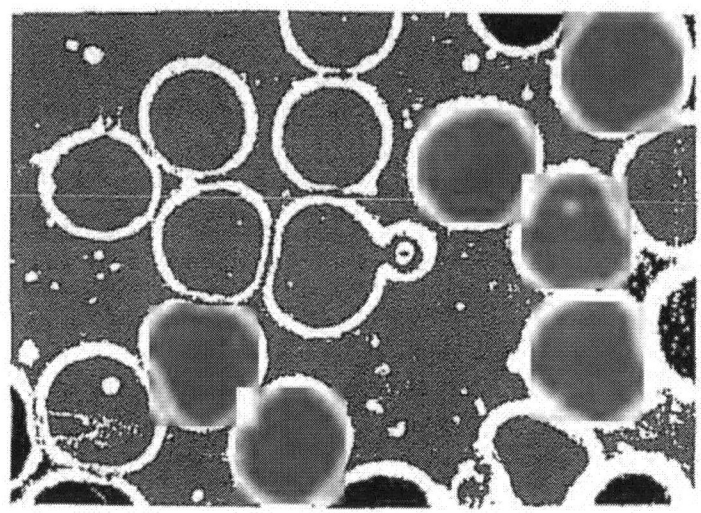

Photograph 20. Just below and to the right of center Is a yeast-like cell ready to separate from the RBC from which it has emerged, the membrane of the JRBC being completely restored, 4,500X.

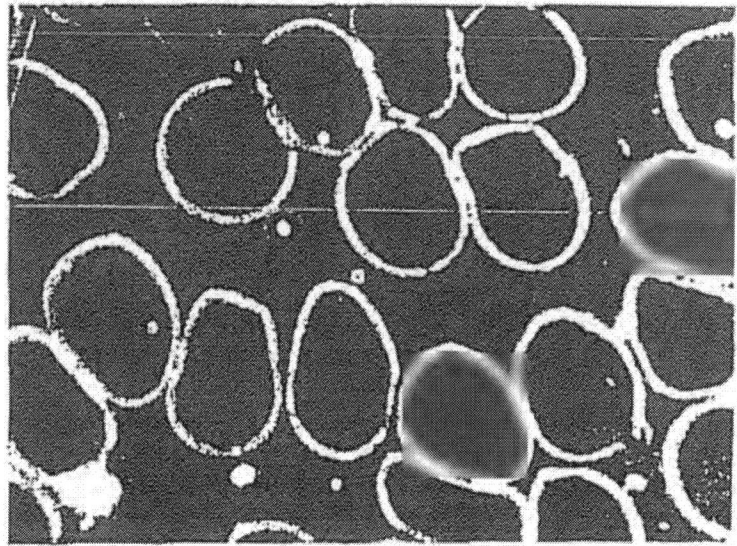

Photograph 21, More budding cells, somatids, spores and double spores in the background, 4,500X.

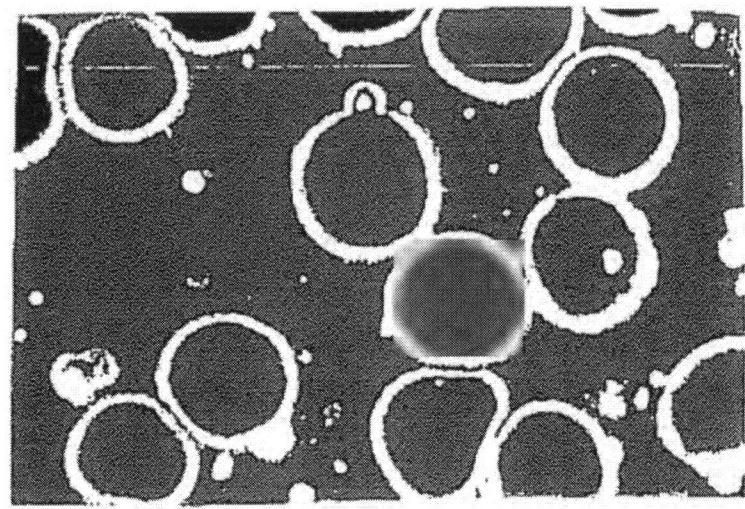

Photograph 22. The blood of pre-cancerous individuals always shows inclusions in some RBCs as seen here. 3,000X.

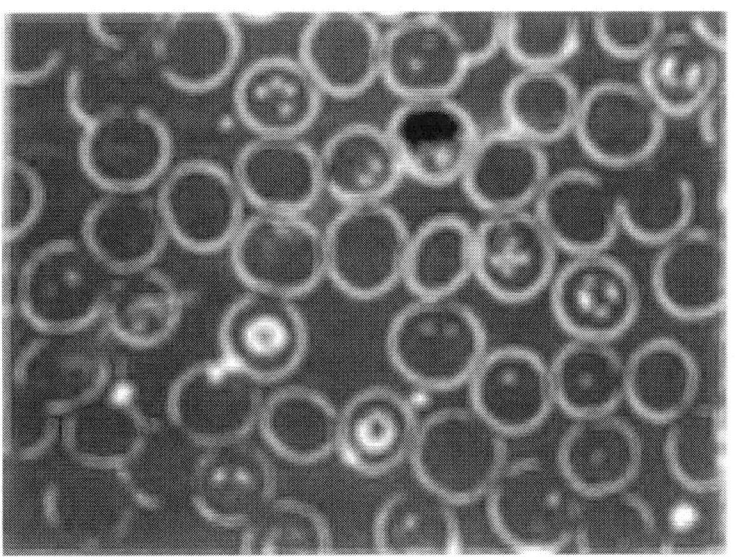

Photograph 23, Increased ration of RBCs having inclusions in an Individual with diagnosed cancer. 3,000X.

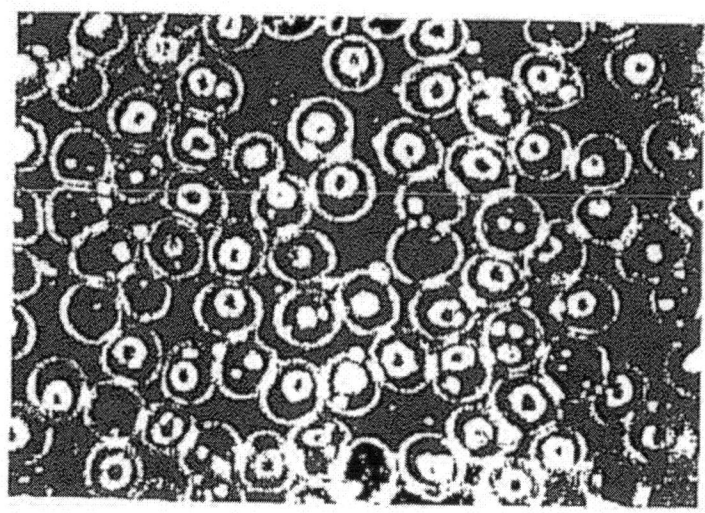

Photograph 24. In terminal cancer all the RBCs show gross Inclusions. 3,000X

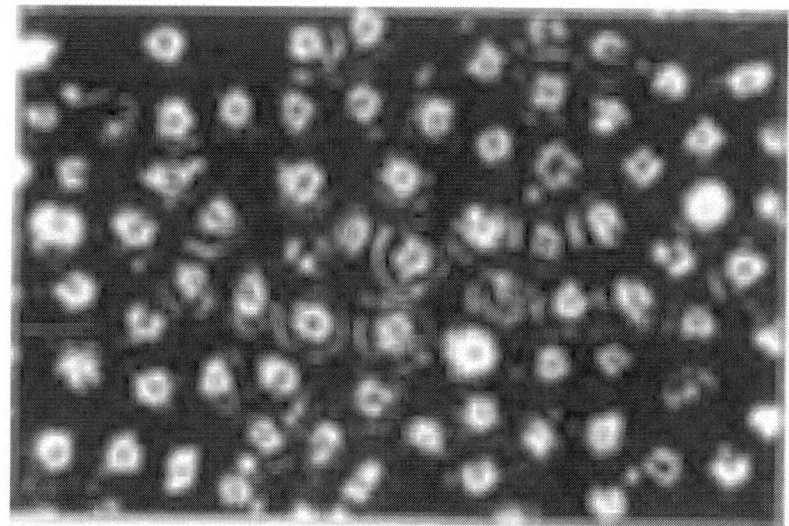

The rate of increase in the number of somatids and other forms in the field appears to be entirely too high to be ascribed to contamination of the saline medium or parasitization of the RBCs.

Viewing this phenomenon directly, or in a time lapse videotape produced by C.E.R.B.E., leaves no doubt that the somatid and other forms originate within the RBCs.

There is a body of belief in hematology having to do with budding or breaking away of fragments of the RBC membrane and with the condensation of hemoglobin into particles or "crystals." These standard hematological observations do not address the phenomenon observed by C.E.R.B.E.

The mature RBC contains no genetic information. Yet when stressed, but not too far removed from in vivo conditions, appears to de-evolve into a variety of living forms.

This phenomenon is not an artifact, i.e. a process induced by the conditions of preparation and observation of the specimen. C.E.R.B.E. has repeatedly demonstrated that in blood

specimens prepared and examined by their method; all processes described in the preceding paragraph are found immediately in the blood of advanced cancer patients but not in the blood of healthy individuals.

There can be no doubt that this disintegration process of the RBC is an ongoing in vivo phenomenon under conditions of disease. Perhaps the better terms with which to attempt to conceptualize this morphological change in the RBC would be de-differentiation or de-evolution.

Certainly, it is not a random disintegration producing a miscellaneous inert residue.

RECENT WORK WITH AIDS AND KAPOSI'S SARCOMA

Examination of the blood, spermatic fluid and tumor tissues from a limited number of individuals having AIDS, or Kaposi's Sarcoma or both, has shown a variety of physiological changes not found in cancer.

The number of specimens examined thus far is not sufficient to confirm the consistency of these observations and no firm conclusions can be drawn as to their meaning or significance. The variety of possible combinations of Kaposi's Sarcoma and opportunistic infections with AIDS presents a highly complex picture.

Photographs 25 through 28 show a pattern of inclusions in lymphocytes and a tendency for this white cell to form conidium heads In Individuals having AIDS only. Photograph 25. Four lymphocytes with inclusions in the nucleus. 4,500X.

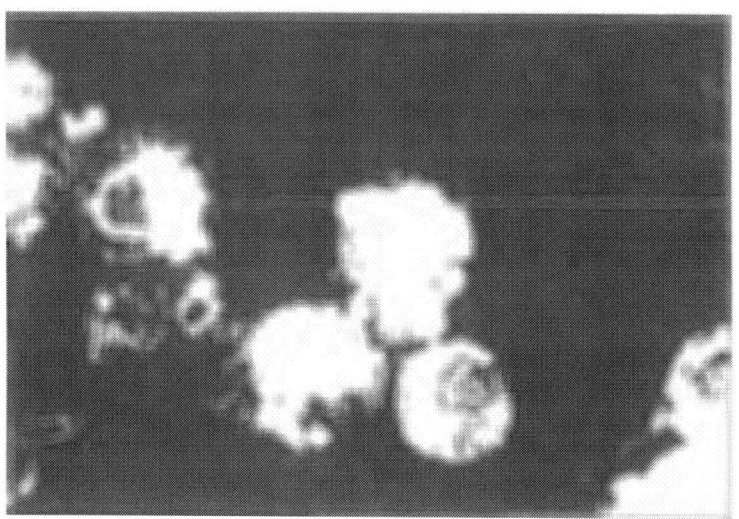

Photograph 26. Next to the large bright cell on the right is a lymphocyte with inclusions. 4,500X. The bright cell has the appearance of a conidium head.

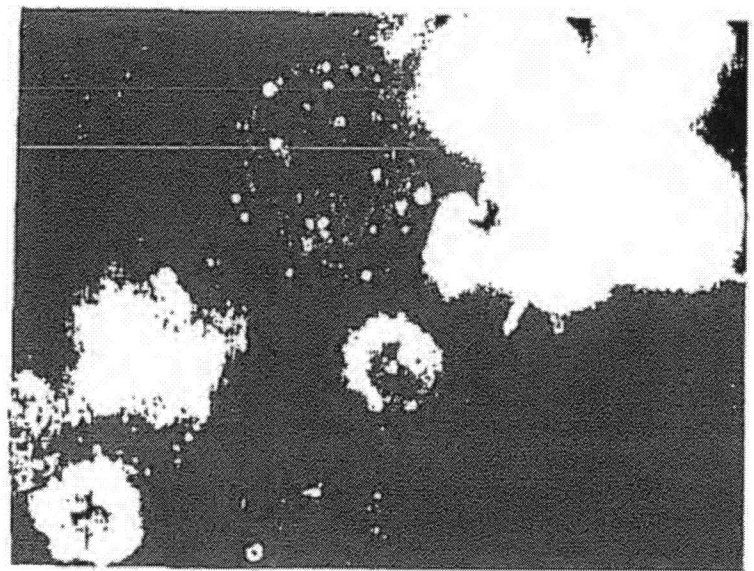

Photograph 27. The dark cell on the right is a lymphocyte with inclusions in the nucleus, 4. S00X. These inclusions are probably a

virus. The large bright form to the left is a conidium head very similar to that of Aspergillus. This may be Important and must be investigated further.

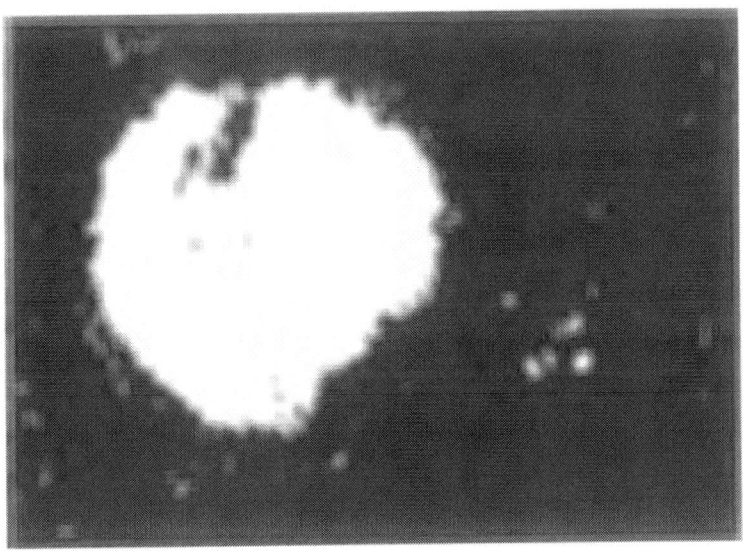

Photograph 28. Another conidium head with many small thalli. A progression from the stage shown in photo 27. 4,500X.

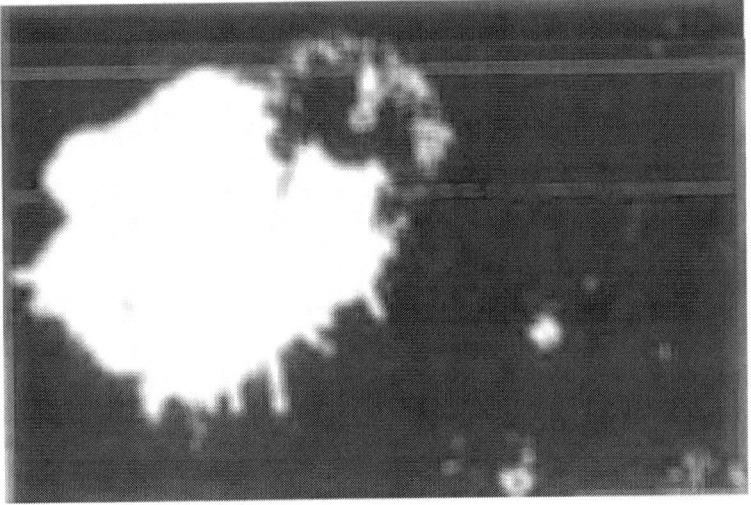

Photographs 29 through 32 show morphologic changes in a large cell, which has some of the features of a monocyte, in blood from an individual having AIDS. Photograph 29. Note the five large inclusions on the right side of the nucleus. 4500X

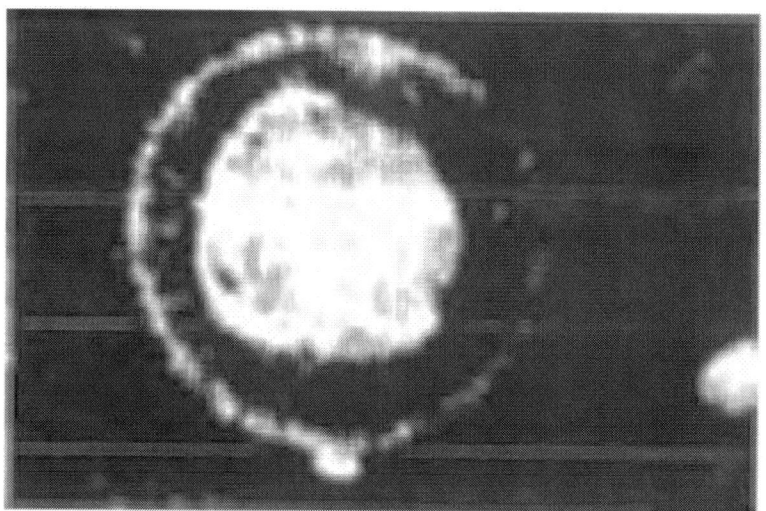

Photograph 30. The same cell ten minutes later, 4,500X. The nucleus Is expanding and the number of visible inclusions is increasing. This is the same magnification as in photo 29, Note the overall increase of the size of this cell.

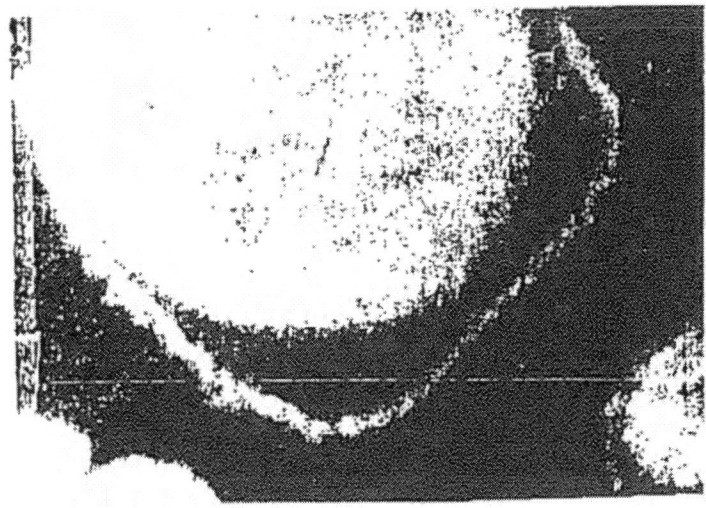

Photograph 31. thirty minutes later (3,500X). Note the external membrane. The nucleus and cytoplasm are swelling.

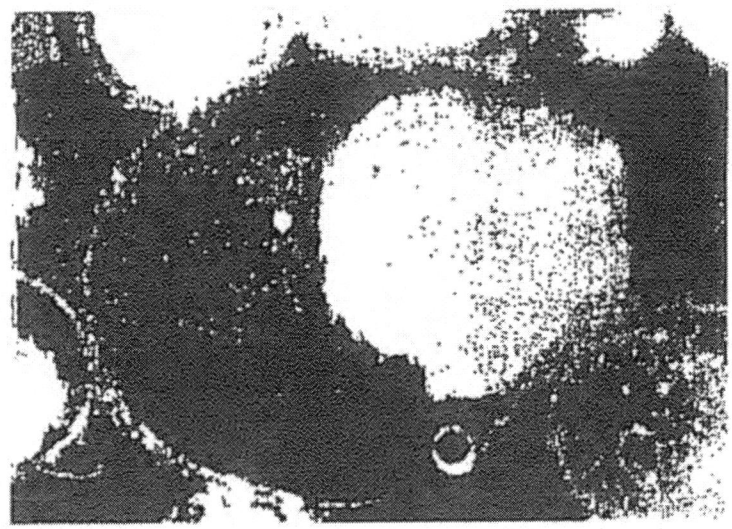

Photograph 32. The same cell after one hour (3,500X). The nucleus occupies the whole cell which will soon burst.

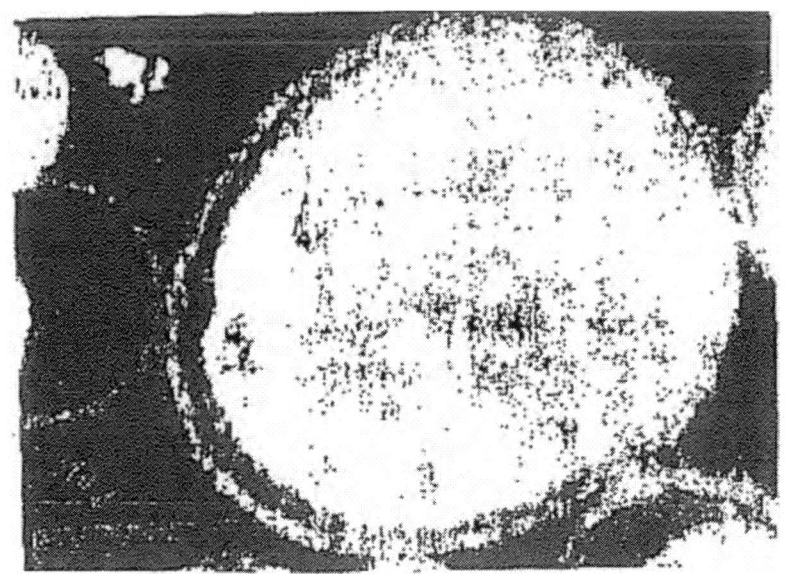

Photos 33 and 34 show Diplococcus and tetrads (groups of four cells) spermatic fluid from two different individuals having AIDS. This appears to be characteristic in AIDS and may be helpful in diagnosis and treatment monitoring. Both photos 3,000X.

Photograph 33.

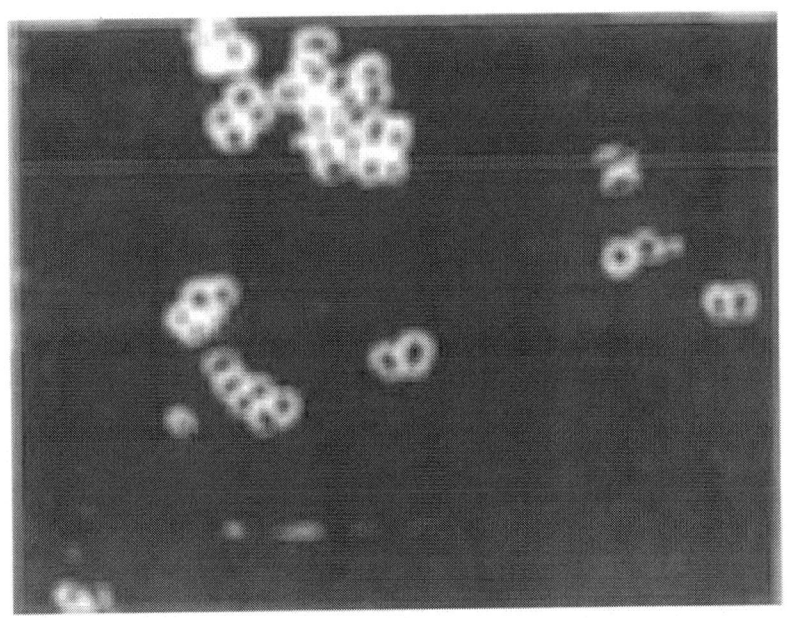

Photograph 34.

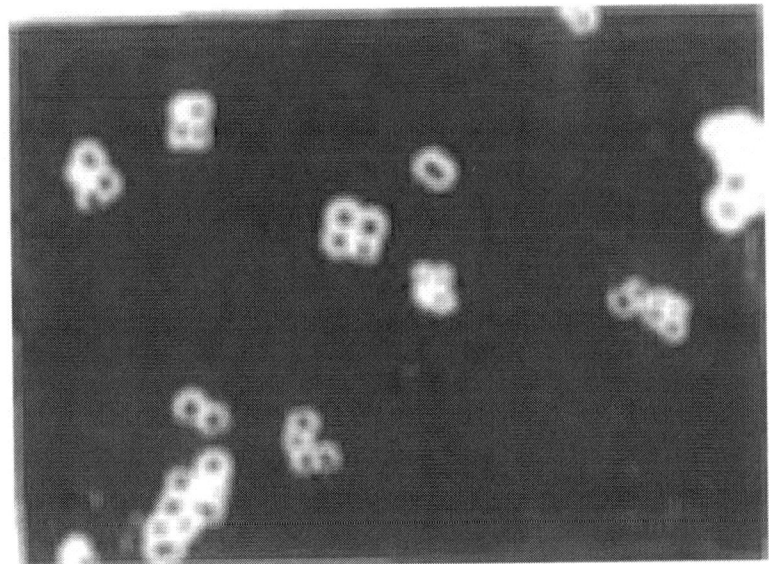

Photos 35 through 42 show the evolution of a characteristic cell found in serum from an individual having AIDS and Kaposi's sarcoma. The serum was transported at 4 degrees centigrade.

Note the round forms and their progression. The specimen is not fixed or stained. These photographs show a living progression in a single sealed slide over a period of 9 days. Two photos were taken each day of observation, approximately 12 hours apart.

Photograph 35-36. First Day. 4,500X.

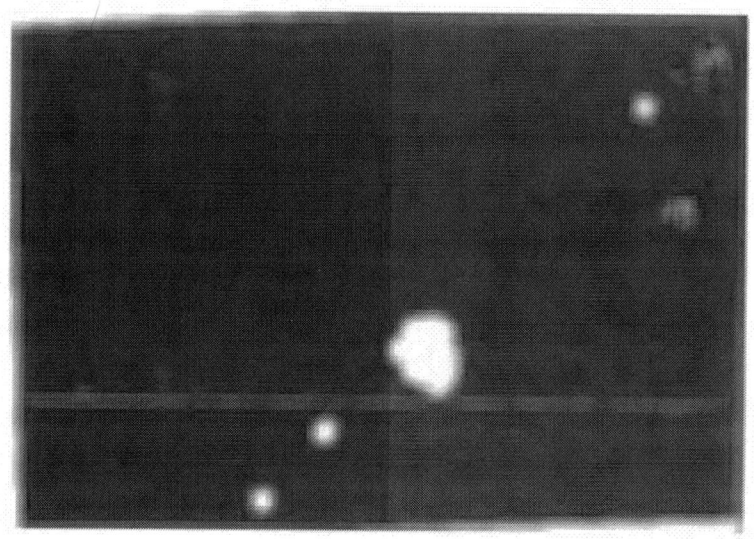

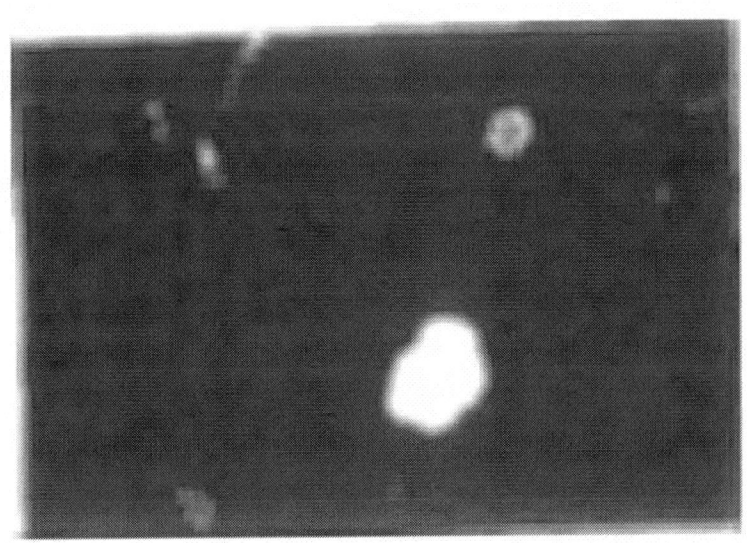

Micrographs 37 through 38. Third day. 4,500X

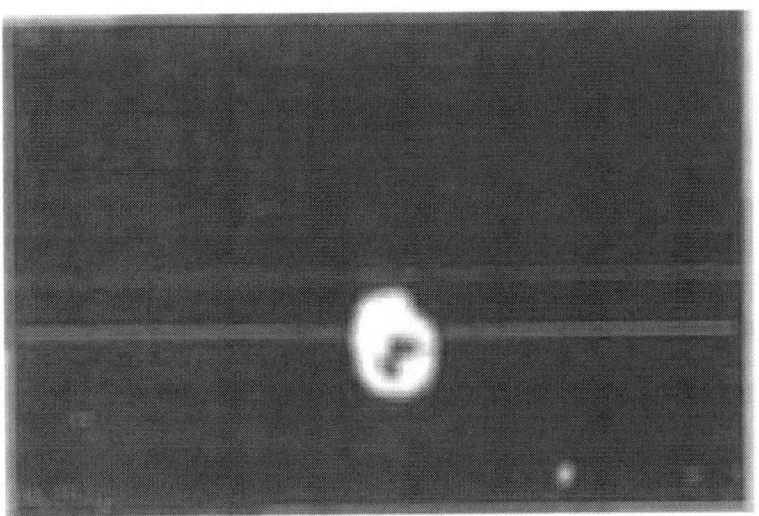

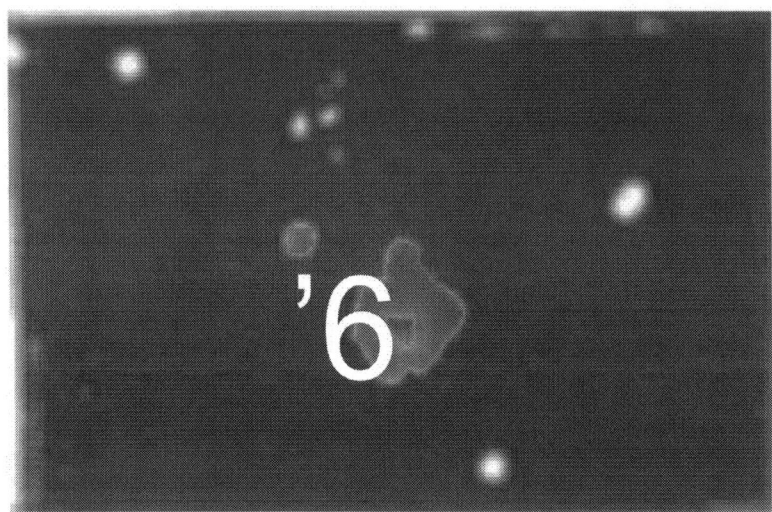

Micrographs 39 through 40, On day five the cell has become larger and contorted, 4,500 X

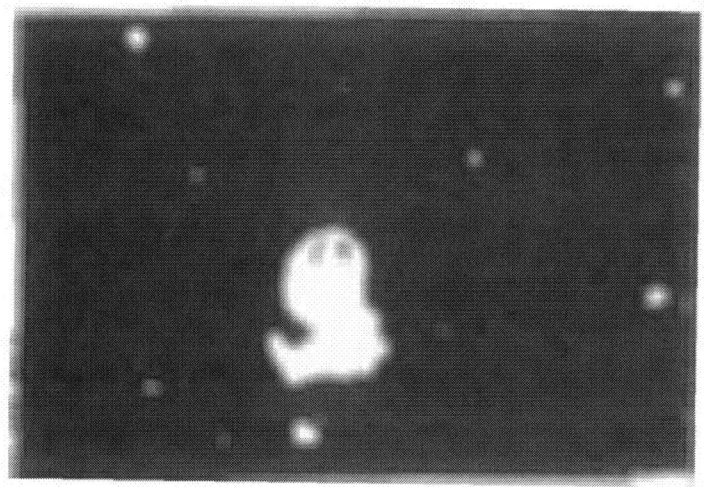

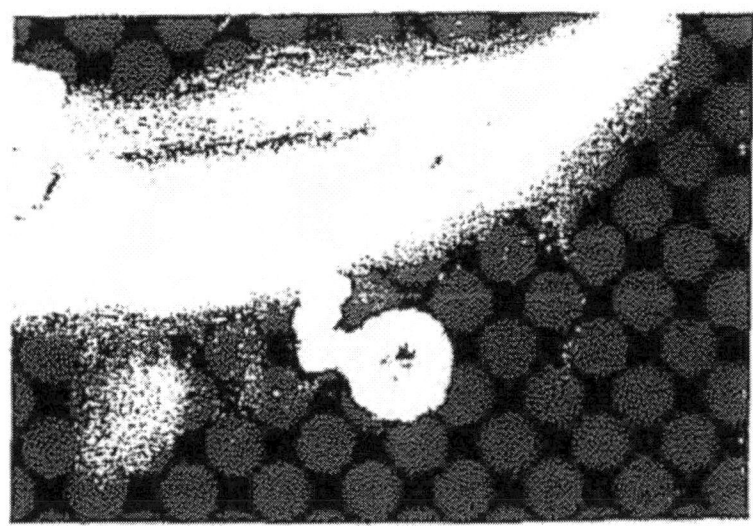

Micrographs 41 through 42. Day nine. In photo 41 the cells appear to be budding and in 42 the large cell has a longer chain configuration as seen also In 39 and 40. Thus far, this kind of formation appears to be characteristic in the serum of Individuals with both AIDS and Kaposi's sarcoma. It has not been seen in other kinds of degenerative diseases.

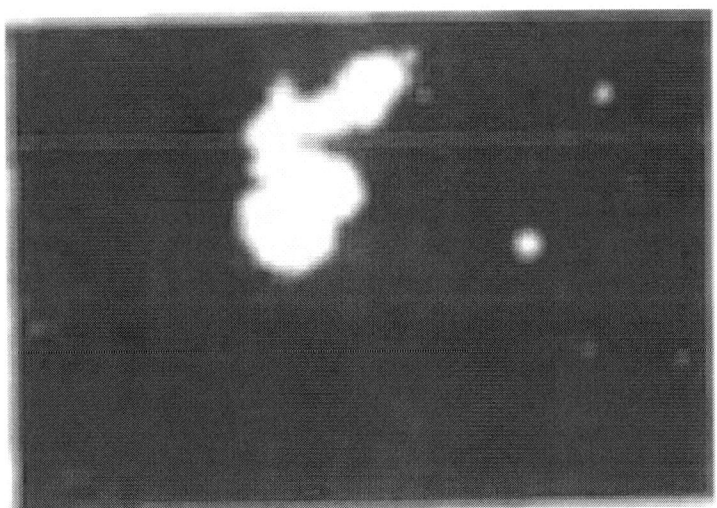

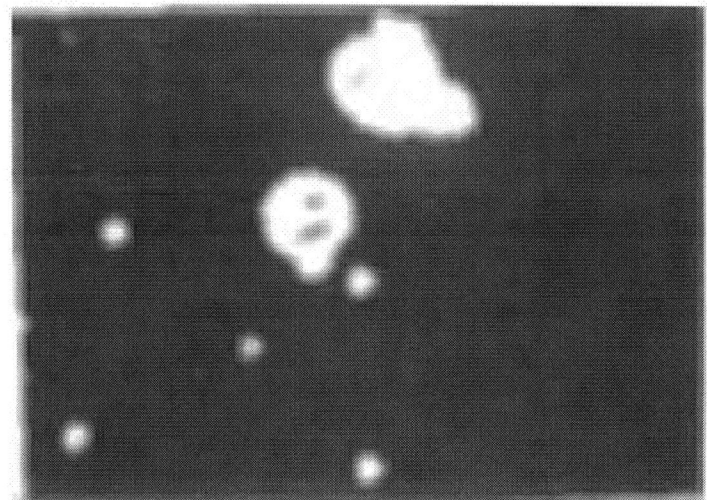

In individuals with both AIDS and Kaposi's sarcoma there appears to be a characteristic problem with integrity of the nucleus of polymorphonuclear cells, as shown by photos 43 and 44.

Photograph 43. The beginning of nuclear division. 4,500X.

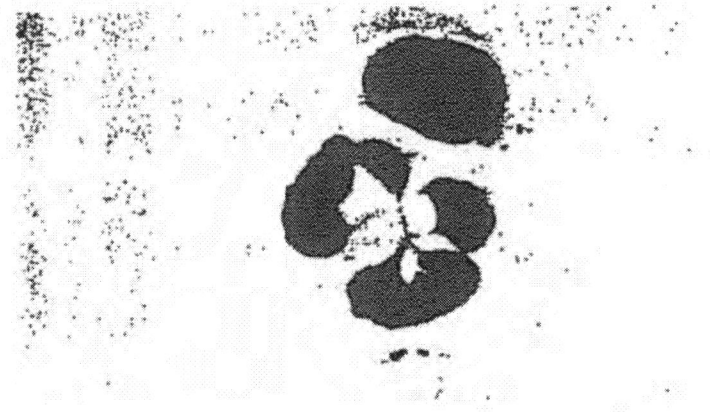

Photograph 44. The same cell 12 hours later (4,500X). The nucleus no longer exists only filaments remain. This kind of transformation

has not been observed in the blood of individuals with classical forms of cancer.

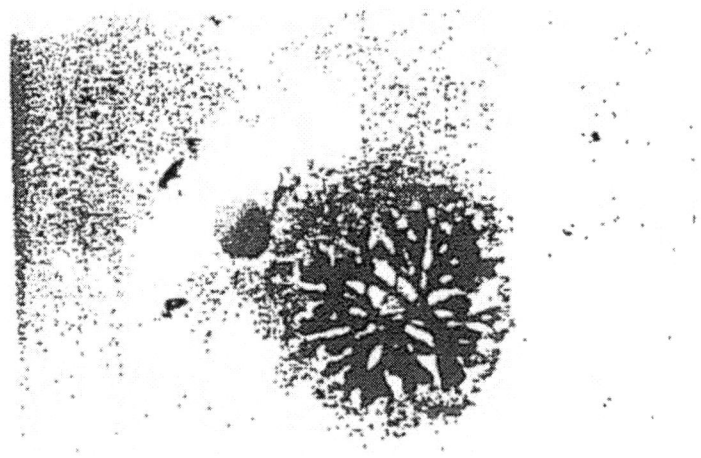

Photographs 45 and 46 show bacterial and fungal activity found in specimens form the tumor of Kaposi's sarcoma.

Photograph 45. Notice the oval shape of the three nuclei (center and upper and lower left) of this tumor cell as well as the filaments at the top. These filaments are characteristic of Kaposi's sarcoma tumor material. Note In particular that the red blood cells do not contain granulations. (4,500X)

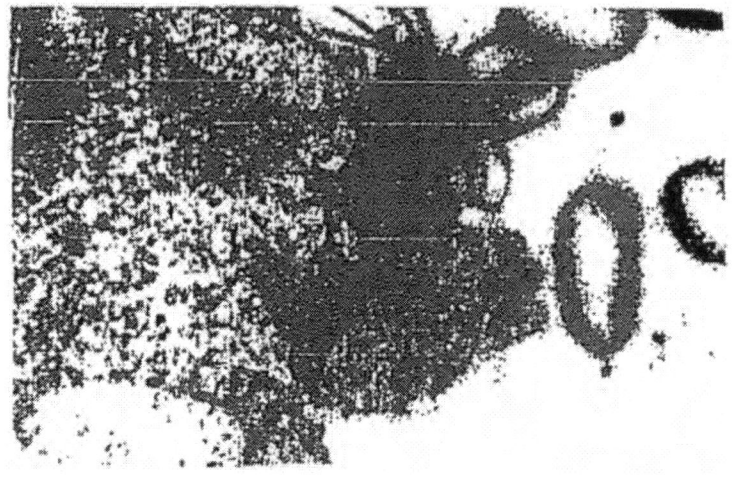

Photograph 46. Same specimen as #45, one hour later. The red cells now contain granulations. (4,500X)

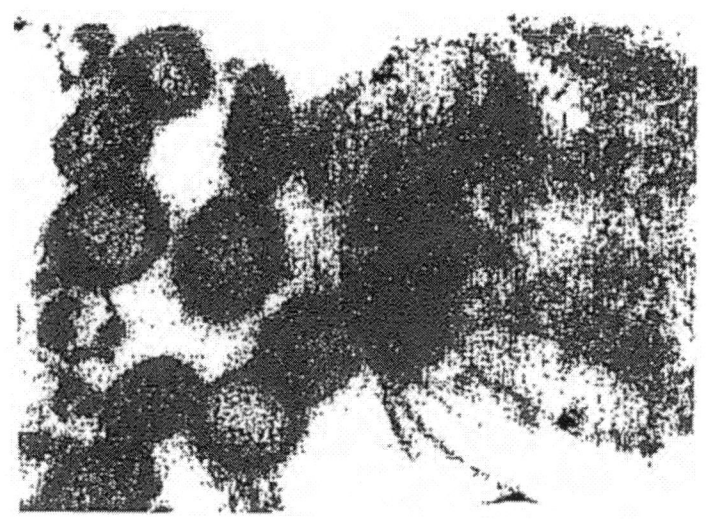

Micrographs 47-54 are of whole blood from inside a Kaposi's tumor.

Photograph 47. Bottom center, fungi and yeast emerging from inside red cells. In the cluster of 6 RBCs on the right, a number of yeast formations. This is always seen in Kaposi tumor material. (4,500X)

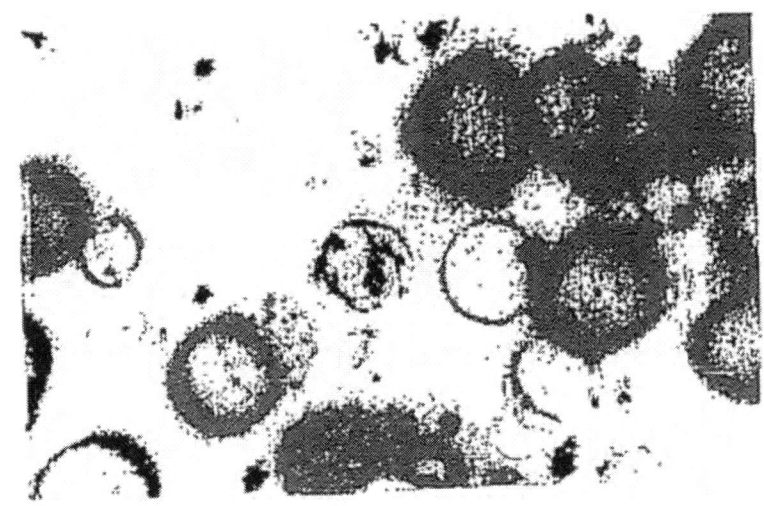

Photograph 48. Note three of the red cells in the upper right contain granulations. (4,500X)

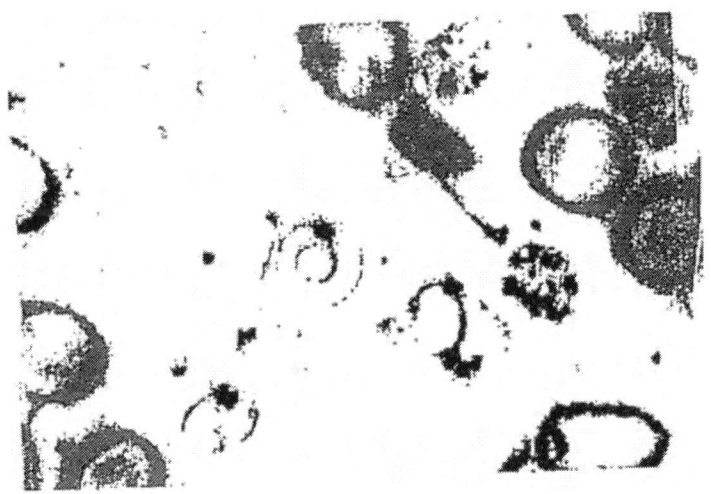

Photograph 49. (4,500X) Just to the left of center a star-shaped configuration has evolved very quickly.

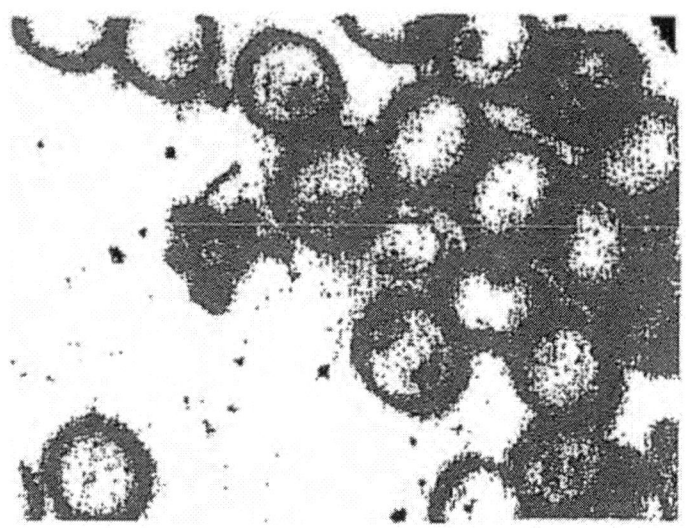

Photograph 50. dog. (4,500X) In the same specimen as in #49 the star-shape has become the caricature of a dog. (4,500X)

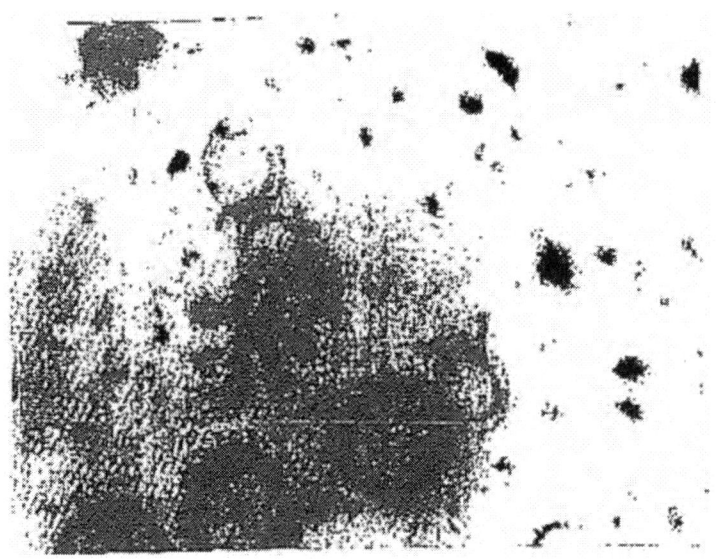

Photograph 51. Filaments forming around a cluster of red cells which have inclusions. (4,500X)

Photograph 52. Mycelia with filaments. (4,500X)

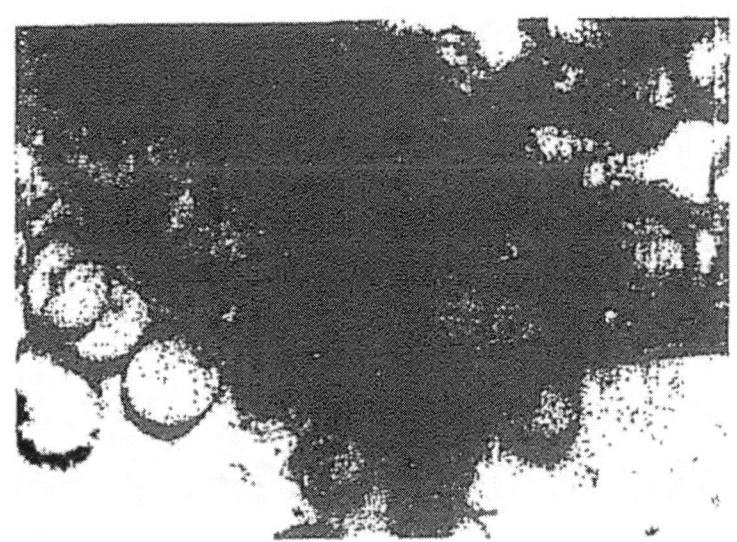

Photograph 53. A large mycelium can be clearly seen here with the ever-present filaments, 4,500X.

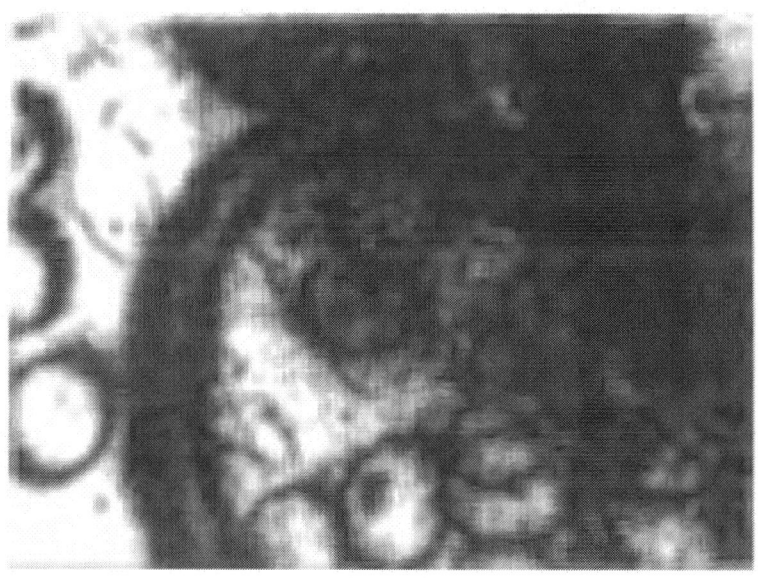

Photograph 54. A closer look at a large mycelium with filaments apparently growing out of it. This specimen is from whole blood of a patient with AIDS and Kaposi's sarcoma. (4,500X).

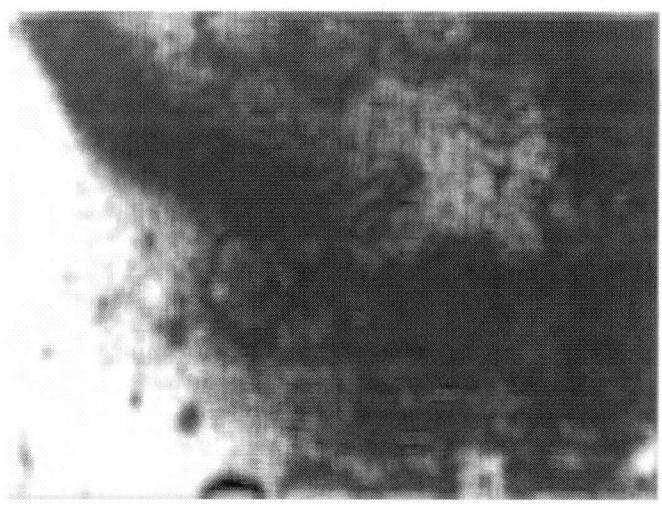

CONCLUSION

Direct observation of grotesque morphological changes in white cells in general suggests current conceptualizations of AIDS and its associated problems are focused too narrowly. While the white cells may be hosting the reproduction of viruses, something of a much greater magnitude appears to be happening.

The white cells are obviously destructing, but the observed end-product is visible quantities of pathogenic bacterial and fungal forms rather than an inert biological waste.

The process generating these forms is associated with the nuclei and is in many ways parallel to those found in the RBCs of cancer. It may be highly significant if further research confirms that in AIDS the white cells evolve pathogenic forms since this phenomenon has been well established by C.E.R.B.E. for the red cells in cancer.

The predominance of filamentous mycelia forms in Kaposi's sarcoma suggests the possibility they may evolve out of the microbial products of white cell nuclei transformations in AIDS. However, the limited number of observations of white cells from individuals having both AIDS and Kaposi's (Photos 43 and 44) show a very different kind of nuclear disturbance from that seen in AIDS only. Al! these forms are distinctly different from those found in cancer.

FOOTNOTES

1. Gaston Naessens, founder and principal investigator.

2. Affiliate professor, Department of Philosophy, Colorado State University, Fort Collins, Colorado 80523.

3. Antoine Bechamp (1816-1908) was among those who opposed the emerging germ theory of disease in the last years of the 19th century. He was a controversial and energetic figure whose published books alone total almost 3,000 pages. The colorful history of Bechamp and his time is interesting and informative, though far too extensive to elaborate upon here. An English translation, by Dr. Montague R. Leverson, M.D., of his last book, The Blood, was published by Boericke & Tafel in 1911.

4. Lynn Margulis and Dorion Sagan, Microcosmos (New York: Summit Books, 1986).

5. Trephone: Carrel, 1924, 1924. Substance used by cells in formation of their protoplasm.

6. W.T. Frankenberger, Jr., "Microbial Production of Bioregulators in Soil" (Sacramento, California Plant and Soil Conference, 1986.)

7. "Plant Hormone in Mammalian Brain'. M.-Th. Le Page-Degivry et al, University of Nice, France. Science news, Vol. 129, No. 13, March 29, 1986.

8. A similar erythrocyte morphology was reported in part by Oliver (3) in 1914 and Kite (4) the same year, by Auer (5) in 1933 and again by Oliver (6) in 1934.

ON THE PARASITIC THEORY OF CANCER

By Gaston Naessens

The fundamental notion of the existence of living corpuscles of a bacterial nature or of microorganisms in the blood of those sick with cancerous or other degenerative diseases, has been upheld by a number of researchers in spite of the fact that this evidence has always been rejected or resisted by scientific authorities and the medical establishment.

The principle stumbling block has been the fact that the diverse observations, described by some researchers, are in fact only the different phases of the polymorphism of a single, fundamental element!

It has been proven for several years that numerous bacteria possess polymorphism, as opposed to the general idea of monomorphism which has existed for many years in scientific research.

If researchers approached the study of bacteriology in cancer with the notion that polymorphism can exist in microorganisms, they would realize that many of the old researchers in cancerous bacteriology were, in fact, on the right path and that their conclusions were correct.

In reviewing the publications of some researchers on the profound causes of cancer, the precise observations and minutiae of description of what the "Pioneers" have called "Parasite," should lend special weight to those who are moving on the same path, and moreover, those men engaged in the preceding research should not be rejected.

In 1851, Rudolph Virchow, described the cancerous cells containing "cavities" of different size and possessing a double membrane. Some of these "cavities" spontaneously divided and revealed a central nucleus containing granules "of the Coccus genus."

Virchow considered these "cavities" as one particular aspect of the cancerous cell and explained the cellular anarchy through the development of this "cavity" in the interior of the mother cell.

In spite of the detailed description of this phenomenon, this important discovery has not gained the attention of the scientific community which considered his observation as an accidental contamination. In 1884, Henry T. Bytlin, President of the College of Surgeons of Great Britain upheld the parasitic theory of cancers.

This theory has been more or less followed by surgeons up to the point where the parasitic theory was discredited by the evidence that malignant tumors derive more or less directly from the normal tissues of the body. It became clear that the parasitic theory of cancer was incorrect.

Recent discoveries on the subject of microorganisms and the part they play in the formation of certain diseases leads us to think that tumorous tissues are not invaded by micro- oganismic parasites but that they contain intrinsic elements having a particular polymorphism.

From 1889 to 1892, the observations of the following came together:

Thomas-Fortschritte der Medicine. #11 Bd. 1889.

Darier-C.R. de la societe de biologie. April 13, 1889.

Malaises--"On the new Psorospermoses of Man," Medicine experimentale et anatomie pahtologique, Tome II, p. 302 ft, 1890.

Nils Sjorbring-Fortschritte der Medicine. "Ein parasitarer protozoartiger organismus in Carcinomen." Bd. Ill #14, p. 529, July 15, 1890.

P. Foa~"Uber die Krebsparasiten," Central blatt fur bacteriologie und Parasitenkunde, Band XII, August 9, 1892.

On December 2, 1890, William Russell, F.R.C.P.E. presents "A characteristic organism of Cancer" to the Pathological Society of London. Layers of cancerous tissues were presented to demonstrate round bodies, hyalins, intra and extra cellular, which he calls "Fushsine Bodies." The "Fushsine Bodies" are round and diverse in size and appear singly or in clusters.

After more in depth studies, Russell classes his organism in the category of fungus or Sprosspilze of Nageli, a class which includes the "Yeast fungus."

In 1890 Louis Wickham describes in "Les Archives de Medicine experimentale et d"Anatomie," Tome II, a "Psorosperme" present in the cells of the nipple in a breast cancer.

On April 13, 1889, Darier, before the Societe de Biologie, demonstrated the presence of a parasite which he named "Psorosperm" in breast cancer.

In March of 1892, Soudakewitch, in the Annales de FInstitut Pasteur, describes a parasite which he encountered in 95 cases of cancer. In August of 1892, he wrote, "The Comparison of all cancer cases observed by myself, confirm my opinion that I was dealing in every case with inclusions of a parasitic nature." The discoveries of Soudakewitch received the backing of eminent zoologists and pathologists.

Metschnikoff declares that the corpuscles described are veritable parasites and not indigenous cellular degenerations. In 1890, Elias Metchnikoff, Department Head at The Pasteur Institute, publishes, "Remarks on carcinomata and coccidia." British Medical Journal, December 10, 1890.

The paper is remarkable in its brilliance and deductive reasoning as well as in the presentation of positive facts in favor of a micro-organism as the cause of cancer.

In 1892, Ruffer and Walker, publish in the Journal de pathologie et Bacteriologie, Volumne I, "On some parasitic Protozoa fotind in cancerous tumors." They give a very detailed observation of cellular inclusions which they considered as true parasites or indigenous cellular formations. They examine many cases of tumors, from all parts of the body, and demonstrated that the parasite is present in each case examined.

They discuss the theory of Klebs and Creighton who suggested that it may be a leucocyte invasion and showed that it is extremely rare to find a leucocyte in a cancerous cell in division.

THE PRIME CAUSE AND PREVENTION OF CANCER

Revised lecture at the meeting of the Nobel-Laureates on June 30, 1966 at Lindau, Lake Constance, GERMANY

By Otto Warburg,

Director, Max Planck-institute for Cell Physiology, Berlin-Dahlem

Preface to the First edition

Motto:

"Why Charles, tell me any good in any new thing. That is excepting Medicine/Winston Churchill to Lord Moran

Most experts agree that nearly 80% of cancers could be prevented, if all contact with the known exogenous carcinogens could be avoided. But how can the remaining 20%, the endogenous or so-called spontaneous cancers, be prevented?

Because no cancer cell exists, the respiration of which is intact, it cannot be disputed that cancer could be prevented if the respiration of the body cells would be kept intact.

Today we know two methods to influence cell respiration. The first is to decrease the oxygen pressure in growing cells. If it is so much decreased that the oxygen transferring enzymes are no longer saturated with oxygen, respiration can decrease irreversibly and normal cells can be transformed into facultative anaerobes. The second method to influence cell respiration in vivo is to add the active groups of the respiratory enzymes to the food of man.

Lack of these groups impairs cell respiration and abundance of these groups repairs impaired cell respiration -- a statement that is proved by the fact that these groups are necessary vitamins for man.

To prevent cancer it is therefore proposed: first to keep the speed of the blood stream so high that the venous blood still contains sufficient oxygen; second, to keep high the concentration of hemoglobin in the blood; third, to add always to the food, even of healthy people, the active groups of these respiratory enzymes and to increase doses of these groups, if a precancerous stated has already developed . If at the same time exogenous carcinogens are excluded rigorously, then much of the endogenous cancer may be prevented today.

These proposals are in no way utopian. On the contrary, they may be realized by everybody, everywhere, at any hour. Unlike the prevention of many other diseases the prevention of cancer requires no government help, and not much money.

Wiesenhof, August 1966 - Otto Warburg

Preface to the Second Edition

Since the Lindau lecture of June 1966 many physicians have examined - not unsuccessfully - the practical consequences of the anaerobiosis of cancer cells. The more who participate in these examinations, the sooner will we know what can be achieved.

It is a unique aspect of these examinations that they can be carried out on human patients, on the largest scale, without notable risk; whereas experiments on animals have been misleading many times; The cure of human cancer will be the resultant of biochemistry of cancer and of biochemistry of man.

A list of selected active groups of respiratory enzymes will soon be published, to which we recently added cytohemin and delta amino Levulinic acid, the precursor of oxygen-transferring hemins.

In the meantime, commercial vitamin preparations may be used that contain, besides other substances, many active groups of the respiratory enzymes. Most of these may be added to the food. Cytohemin and vitamin B 12 may be given subcutaneously. (A synonym of "active group" is "prosthetic" group of an enzyme.)

There exists no alternative today [ed. note, this was 1966, before we had recognized the work of Naessens and others] to the prevention of cancer as proposed at Lindau. It is the way that attacks the prime cause of cancer most directly and that is experimentally most developed.

Indeed, millions of experiments in man, through the effectiveness of some vitamins, have shown, that cell respiration is impaired if the active groups of the respiratory enzymes are removed from the food; and that cell respiration is repaired at once, if these groups are added again to the food.

No way can be imagined that is scientifically better founded to prevent and cure a disease, the prime cause of which is an impaired respiration. Neither genetic codes of anaerobiosis nor general cancer viruses are alternatives today, because no such codes and no such viruses in man have been discovered so far; but anaerobiosis has been discovered.

What can be achieved by the active groups, when tumors have already developed? The answer is doubtful, because tumors live in the body almost anaerobically, that is under conditions that active groups cannot act.

On the other hand, because young metastases live in the body almost aerobically, inhibition by the active groups should be possible. Therefore, we propose first to remove all compact tumors, which are anaerobic foci of the metastases.

Then the active groups should be added to the food in the greatest possible amount, for many years, even for ever. This is a promising task. If it succeeds, then cancer will be a harmless disease.

Moreover, we discovered recently* in experiments with growing cancer cells in vitro, that very low concentrations of some selected active groups inhibit fermentation and growth of cancer cells completely, in the course of a few days. From these experiments it may be concluded that de-differentiated cells die if one tries to normalize their metabolism.

It is a result that is expected and that encourages the task of inhibiting the growth of metastases with active enzyme groups, As emphasized, it is the first precondition of the proposed treatment that al! growing body cells be saturated with oxygen.

It is a second precondition that exogenous carcinogens be kept away, at least during the treatment. All carcinogens impair respiration directly or indirectly by deranging capillary circulation, a statement that is proved by the fact that no cancer cell exists, the respiration of which is not impaired. Of course, respiration cannot be repaired if it is impaired at the same time by carcinogens.

It has been asked after the Lindau lecture why repair of respiration by the active groups of enzymes was proposed as late as 1966, although the fermentation of the cancer cells was discovered as early as 1923. Why was so much time lost? He who asked this question ignored that in 1923 the chemical mechanism of enzyme action was still a secret of living nature alone.1 The first active group of an enzyme, "Iron, the Oxygen-Transferring Part of the Respiratory Enzyme" was discovered in 1924.

There followed in two decades the discoveries of the hemoproteins, the flavoproteins and the pyridinproteins, a period that was concluded by the "Heavy Metals as a Prosthetic Group of Enzymes"3 and by the "Hydrogen Transferring Enzymes" A in 1947 to 1949,

Moreover, during the first decades after 1923 glycolysis and anaerobiosis were constantly confused, so nobody knew what was specific for tumors. The three famous and decisive discoveries of Dean Burk and colleagues3 of the National Cancer. Institute at Bethesda were of the years 1941, 1956 and 1964:

first, that the metabolism of the regenerating liver, which grows more rapidly than most tumors, is not cancer metabolism, but perfect aerobic embryonic metabolism;

second, that cancer cells, descended in vitro from one single normal cell, were in vivo the more malignant, the higher the fermentation rate;

third, that in vivo growing hepatomas, produced in vivo by different carcinogens, were in vivo the more malignant, the higher the fermentation rate.

Furthermore, the very unexpected and fundamental fact, that tissue culture is carcinogenic and that a too low oxygen pressure is the intrinsic cause, were discovered3"3 in the years 1927 to 1966. Anaerobiosis of cancer cells was an established fact only since 1960, when methods were developed 7 to measure the oxygen pressure inside of tumors in the living body.

This abridged history shows that even the greatest genius would not have been able to propose in 1923, what was proposed at Lindau in 1966. As unknown as the prime cause of cancer was in 1923 was the possibility to prevent it.

Life without oxygen in a living world that has been created by oxygen9 was so unexpected that it would have been too much to ask that anaerobiosis of cancer cells should be accepted at once by all scientists.

But most of the resistance disappeared when at Lindau it was explained that on the basis of anaerobiosis there is now a real chance to get rid of this terrible disease, if man is willing to submit to experiments and facts. It is true that more than 40 years were necessary to learn how to do it. But 40 years is a short time in the history of science.

Wiesenhof uber Idar-Oberstein, August 1967, Otto Warburg

The Prime Cause and Prevention of Cancer

There are prime and secondary causes of diseases. For example, the prime cause of the plague is the plague bacillus, but secondary causes of the plague are filth, rats, and the fleas that transfer the plague bacillus from rats to man. By prime cause of a disease I mean one that is found in every case of the disease.

Cancer above all other diseases, has countless secondary causes. Almost anything can cause cancer. But even for cancer there is only one prime cause.

Summarized in a **few** words: **The prime cause of cancer is the replacement of the respiration of oxygen in normal body cells by a fermentation of sugar.** All normal body cells meet their energy needs by respiration of oxygen whereas cancer cells meet their energy needs in great part by fermentation.

All normal body cells are thus obligate aerobes, whereas all cancer cells are partial anaerobes. From the standpoint of the physics and chemistry of life this difference between normal and cancer cells is so great that one can scarcely picture a greater difference.

Oxygen gas, the donor of energy in plants and animals is dethroned in the cancer cells, and replaced by an energy yielding reaction of the lowest living forms, namely, a fermentation of glucose.

The key to the cancer problem is accordingly the energetics of life, which has been the field of work in the Dahlem institute since its initiation by the Rockefeller Foundation about 1930. In Dahlem the oxygen transferring and hydrogen transferring enzymes were discovered and chemically isolated.

In Dahlem the fermentation of cancer cells was discovered decades ago; but only in recent years has it been demonstrated that cancer cells can actually grow in the body almost with only the energy of fermentation.

Only today can one submit, with respect to cancer, all the experiments demanded by Pasteur and Koch as proof of the prime cause of a disease. If it is true that the replacement of oxygen-respiration by fermentation is the prime cause of cancer, then all cancer cells without exception must ferment, and no normal growing cell ought to exist that ferments in the body.

An especially simple and convincing experiment performed by the Americans Malmgren and Flanegan confirms this view. If one injects tetanus spores, which can germinate only at very low oxygen pressures, into the blood of healthy mice, the mice do not sicken with tetanus, because the spores find no place in the normal body where the oxygen pressure is sufficiently low.

Likewise, pregnant mice do not sicken when injected with tetanus spores, because also in the growing embryo no region exists where the oxygen pressure is sufficiently low to permit spore germination.

However, if one injects tetanus spores into the blood of tumor-bearing mice, the mice sicken with tetanus, because the oxygen pressure in the tumors can be so low that the spores germinate. These experiments demonstrate in a unique way the anaerobiosis of cancer cells and the non-anaerobiosis of normal cells, and in particular the non-anaerobiosis of normal growing embryos.

THE FERMENTATION OF MORRIS HEPATOMAS

A second type of experimentation demonstrates a quantitative connection between fermentation of tumors and growth rate of tumors.

If one injects rats with cancer-inducing substances of different activities, one can create, as Harold Morris of the National Cancer Institute of Bethesda has found, liver cancers (hepatomas) of very different degrees of malignancy. Thus, one strain of tumor may double its mass in three days, another strain may require 30 days.

Recently Dean Burk and Mark Woods also of the National Cancer Institute, measured the in vitro rates of anaerobic fermentation in different lines of these hepatomas, and obtained a curve (Fig. 1) that shows a quantitative relationship between fermentation and growth rate, and therefore between fermentation and malignancy, in these various tumor strains. The fermentation increases with the malignancy, and indeed the fermentation increases even faster than the malignancy.

Special interest attaches to the fermentation of the most slowly growing hepatomas, because several investigators in the United States believed that they found that such tumors had no fermentation, which would have meant that there can-be tumors growing without fermentation; that is, that anaerobiosis cannot be the prime cause of cancer.

Fig. I Velocity of growth and fermentation of Morris Hepatomas, according to Dean Burk and Mark Woods.

Dean Burk and Mark Woods saw immediately from their curves that in the region of the zero point the rate of fermentation was so small that it could no longer be measured by the usual gross methodology employed by the aforementioned workers, whereas in the same region the smallest growth rate was always easily measurable. Burk and Woods saw in other words, that in the region of the zero point of their curves the growth test was more sensitive than the usual fermentation test.

With refined and adequate methods for measuring fermentation of sugar (glucose) they found, what any physical chemist after a glance at the curve would realize, that even the most slow-growing Morris hepatomas fermented sugar.

The results of Dean Burk and Mark Woods were confirmed and extended by other workers with other independent methods. Pietro Gullino, also in Bethesda, developed a perfusion method whereby a Morris hepatoma growing in the living animal could be perfused for long periods of time, even weeks, by means of a single artery and single vein, and the blood entering and leaving any given tumor could be analyzed.

Gullino found with this method that the slow-growing Morris hepatomas always produced fermentation lactic acid during their growth. This was in contrast to liver, where, as known since the days of Claude Bernard, lactic acid is not produced but consumed by liver; the difference between liver and Morris tumors in vitro is thus infinite (+ vs. -).

Gullino further found that tumors grow in vivo with diminished oxygen consumption. In summary, Gullino's findings indicate that the slow-growing Morris hepatomas are partial anaerobes.

Silvio Fiala, a biochemist at the University of Southern California, found that not only did the slow-growing hepatomas produce lactic acid, but also the number of their oxygen-respiring grana was reduced.

The slow-growing Morris hepatomas are therefore far removed from having refuted the tumors. On the contrary they are the best proof of this distinctive characteristic.

For over forty years cancer investigators have searched for a cancer that did not ferment.

Additionally, a non-fermenting tumor appeared to have been found in the slow-growing Morris tumors, it was soon shown to be a methodological error.

TRANSFORMATION OF EMBRYONIC METABOLISM INTO CANCER METABOLISM

A third type of experiment, from the institute in Dahlem with co-workers Gawehn, Geissler and Lorenz, is likewise highly pertinent.

Having established that anaerobiosis is that property of cancer cells that distinguishes them from all normal body cells, we then attacked the next question, namely, how normal body cells can become transformed into cancer cells.

If one puts embryonic mouse cells into a suitable culture medium saturated with physiological oxygen pressures, they will grow outside the mouse body, in vitro, and indeed as pure aerobes, with a pure oxygen respiration, without a trace of fermentation.

However, if during the growth one provides an oxygen pressure so reduced that the oxygen respiration is partially inhibited, the purely aerobic metabolism of the mouse embryonic cells is quantitatively altered within 48 hours, in the course of two cell divisions, into the metabolism characteristic of fermenting cancer cells. Fig. 2 illustrates the very simple experimental procedure involved.

If one then brings such cells, in which during their growth under reduced oxygen pressure a cancer cell metabolism has been produced, back under the original high pressure, the cancer metabolism remains.

The transformation of embryonic cell metabolism into cancer cell metabolism can thus be irreversible, an important result, since the origin of cancer cells from normal body cells is itself an irreversible process.

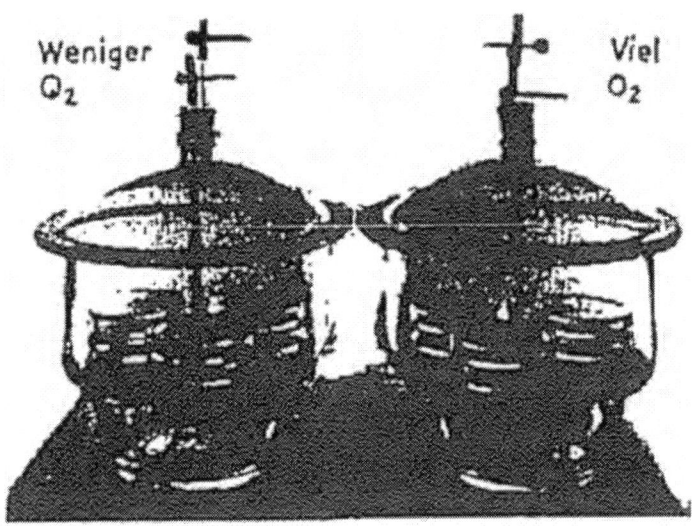

Fig. 2 Method to transform embryonic metabolism into cancer metabolism by decreasing the oxygen pressure.

It is equally important that these body cells whose metabolism has thus been transformed into cancer metabolism now continue to grow in vitro as facultative anaerobes. The duration of our experiments is still too limited to have yielded results of tests of inoculation of such cells back into mice, but according to all previous indications such cells will later grow as anaerobes upon transplantation into animals.

in any case, these experiments belong to the most important experiments in the field of cancer investigation since the discovery of the fermentation of tumors. For cancer metabolism, heretofore measured so many thousands of times, has now been induced artificially in body cells by the simplest conceivable experimental procedure, and with this artificially induced cancer metabolism the body cells divide and grow anaerobes in vitro.

In recent months we have further developed our experimental arrangements so that we can measure monometrically the oxygen respiration and fermentation of the growing mouse embryonic cells during the metabolic transformation.

Fig. 3 shows the experimental arrangement. We find by such experiments that 35 percent inhibition of oxygen respiration already suffices to bring about such a transformation during cell growth. *

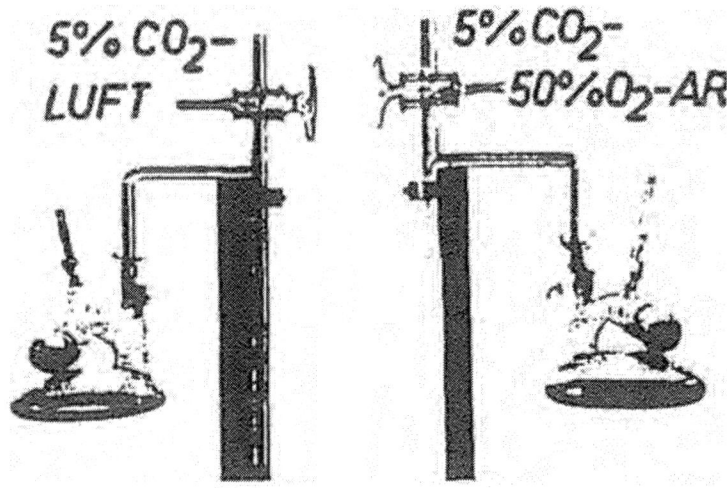

Fig. 3 Method to measure manometrically respiration and fermentation during the transformation of embryonic into cancer metabolism. *

Oxygen pressures that inhibit respiration 35 percent can occur at the ends of blood capillaries in living animals, so that the possibility arises that cancer may result when too low oxygen pressures occur during cell growth in animal bodies.

The induction of cancers by solid materials injected into animals is a further experimental indication of this possibility.

If one implants discs of solid substances under the skin of rats, the discs will soon be surrounded by capsules of living tissue that will be nourished with blood vessels from the hypodermis. Sarcomas very frequently develop in these capsules.

It is immaterial whether the solid discs are chemically plastics, gold, or ivory, etc. What produces the cancer is not the chemical nature of the sold discs, but the special kind of blood provision varies with the site and in adequacy within a given animal, and induces cancer from the low oxygen pressure in the encapsulating disc.

THERMODYNAMICS

If now a lowered oxygen pressure during cell growth may cause cancer, or, more generally, if any inhibition of respiration during growth may cause cancer, then a next problem is to show why reduced respiration induces cancer.

Since we already know that with a lowering of respiration fermentation results, we can re- express our question: Why does cancer result if oxygen-respiration is replaced by fermentation? To answer this question, we must go back to the early history of life. **

The early history of life on our planet indicates that life existed on earth before the earth's atmosphere contained free oxygen gas. The living cells must therefore have been fermenting cells then, and, as fossils show, they were undifferentiated single cells.

Only when free oxygen appeared in the atmosphere -- some billion years ago - did the higher development of life set in, to produce the plant and animal kingdoms from the fermenting, undifferentiated single cells. What philosophers of life have called "Evolution creatrice" is therefore the work of oxygen.

The reverse process, the dedifferentiation of life, takes place today in greatest amount before our eyes in cancer development, which is another expression for dedifferentiation.

To be sure, cancer development takes place even in the presence of free oxygen gas in the atmosphere, but this oxygen may not penetrate in sufficient quantity into the growing body cells, or the respiratory enzymes of the growing body cells may be damaged.

In any case, during the cancer development the oxygen-respiration always falls, fermentation appears, and the highly differentiated cells are transformed to fermenting anaerobes, which have lost all their body functions and retain only the now useless property of growth.

Thus, when respiration disappears, life does not disappear, but the meaning of life disappears, and what remains are growing machines that destroy the body in which they grow. From these facts the next question arises: why oxygen differentiates and lack of oxygen dedifferentiates?

Nobody would dispute that the development of plants and animals and man from unicellular anaerobes is the most improbable process of all processes in the world.

But according to the thermodynamics of Boltzmann, improbable processes require work to take place. It requires work to produce temperature differences in a uniformly temperatured gas; whereas the equalization of such temperature differences is a spontaneous process that does not require work.

It is the oxygen-respiration that provides in life this work, and dedifferentiation begins at once when respiration is inhibited in any way.

In the language of thermodynamics, differentiation represents a forced steady state, whereas dedifferentiation - that is, cancer -- is the true equilibrium state.

Or, illustrated by a picture: the differentiated body cell is like a ball on an inclined plane, which would roll down except for the work of oxygen-respiration always preventing this.

If oxygen-respiration is inhibited, the ball rolls down the plane to the level of dedifferentiation. But one fact can still not be explained by physics: why the work of respiratory energy and not that of fermentation energy can differentiate, whereas in general, for example in growth, respiratory energy and fermentation energy are equivalent.

Obviously, there would be no cancer if there were not this discrimination of fermentation energy, that is, if fermentation like respiration could differentiate.

Then, when respiration is replaced by fermentation, fermentation would take over differentiation, and a high state of differentiation would be maintained in the fermenting body cells.

CHEMISTRY

Physics cannot explain why the two kinds of energy are not equivalent in differentiation; but chemistry may explain it. Biochemists know that both respiration energy and fermentation energy do their work as phosphate energy, but the ways of phosphorylation are different.

If one applies this knowledge to carcinogenesis, it seems that only oxidative phosphorylation but not fermentative phosphorylation can differentiate, a result that may some day explain the mechanism of differentiation.

Yet Biochemistry can explain today why fermentation arises, when respiration decreases. Figure. 4 shows that the pathways of respiration and fermentation are common as far as pyruvic acid. Then the pathways diverge.

The end product of fermentation is reached by one single reaction, the reduction of pyruvic acid by dihydro-nicotinamide to lactic acid.

On the other hand, the end products of the oxidation of pyruvic acid, H2O and CO2, are only reached by 30 additional reactions. Therefore, when cells are harmed, it is most probable that the respiration is harmed.

In this way the frequency of cancer is explained by reasons of probability.

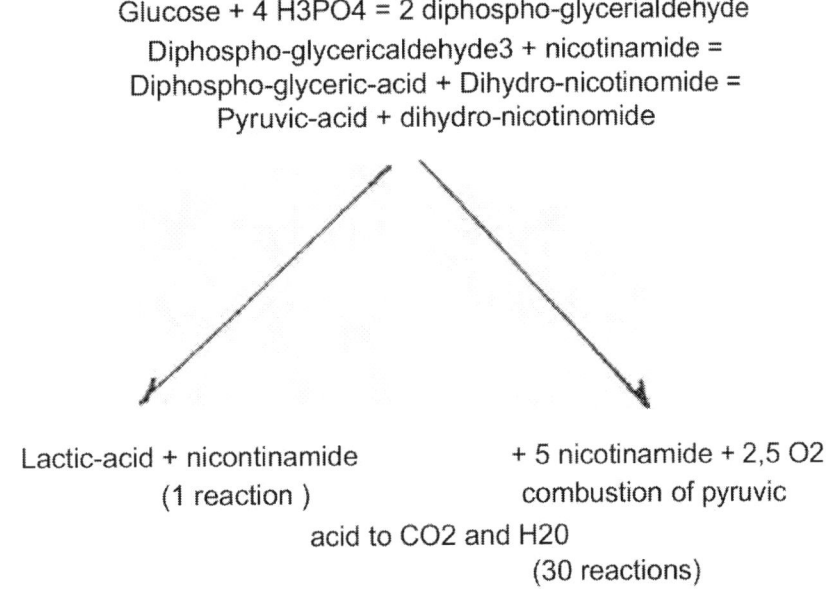

Figure 4

To sum up:

1. Impairment of respiration is frequent, because respiration is more complicated than fermentation.

2. The impaired respiration is replaced by fermentation, because both processes have a common catalyst, the nicotinamide.

3. The consequence of the replacement of respiration by fermentation is mostly glycolysis, with death of the cells by lack of energy. Only if the energy of fermentation is equivalent to the lost energy of respiration, is the consequence anaerobiosis. Glycolysis means death by fermentation, anaerobiosis means life by fermentation.

4. Cancer then arises, because respiration but not fermentation, can maintain and create the high differentiation of body cells.

To conclude the discussion the prime cause of cancer, the virus-theory of cancer may be mentioned. It is the most cherished topic of the philosophers of cancer.

If it were true, then it would be possible to prevent and cure cancer by the methods of virology; and all carcinogens could be eaten or smoked freely without any danger, if only contact with the virus would be avoided.

It is true that some virus-caused cancers* occur in animals but no one sure human virus- cancer has been observed so far, whereas innumerable substances cause cancer without viruses in animals and man.

Thus, viruses do not meet the demands of Pasteur, that it must be possible to trace the prime cause in every case of the disease. Therefore, science classifies viruses as remote causes of cancer, leading to anaerobiosis, the prime case that meets the demands of Pasteur.

Many may remember how anaerobiosis as prime cause of cancer was recently disputed emphatically, when one single cancer - the slow Morris hepatomas - was believed (wrongly) to lack in fermentation.

In contrast, the virus theory is adhered to although almost all cancers of man are lacking in virus-origin. This means the surrender of the principles of Pasteur and the relapse into bygone times of medicine.

APPLICATIONS

Of what use is it to know the prime cause of cancer? Here is an example. In Scandinavian countries there occurs a cancer of the throat and oesophagus whose precursor is the so-called Plummer-Vinson syndrome.

This syndrome can be healed when one adds to the diet the active groups of respiratory enzymes, for example: iron salts, riboflavin, nicotinamide, and pantothenic acid. When one can heal the precursor of cancer, one can prevent cancer.

According to Ernest Wynder of Sloan-Kettering Institute for Cancer Research in New York, the time has come when one can exterminate this kind of cancer with the help of the active groups of the respiratory enzymes.

It is of interest in this connection that with the help of one of these active groups of the respiratory enzymes, namely nicotinamide, tuberculosis can be healed quite well as with streptomycin, but without the side effects of the latter.

Since sulfonamides and antibiotics, this discovery made in 1945 is the most important event in the field of chemotherapy generally, and encourages, in association with the experiences in Scandinavia, efforts to prevent cancer by dietary addition of large amounts of active groups of the respiratory enzymes. Since there can scarcely be over dosage, such experiments can do no harm.

I would like to go further and propose always making dietary additions of large amounts of the active groups of the respiratory enzymes after successful operations when there is danger from metastatic growths. One could indeed never succeed in dedifferentiating the dedifferentiated cancer cells, since during the short duration of human life the probability of such a back-differentiation is zero.

But one might increase the respiration of living metastases, and thereby inhibit their fermentation, and -- on the basis of the curve of Dean Burk and Mark Woods obtained with the Morris hepatomas -- thereby inhibit the growth of metastases to such an extent that they might become as harmless as the so-called "sleeping" cancer cells in the prostates of elderly men.

A SECOND EXAMPLE OF APPLICATION

The physicist Manfred von Ardenne has recently applied his great technical skill to the therapy of cancer. Von Ardenne starts with the general observation that cancer cells are usually more sensitive to high temperatures than are normal cells.

On this basis, he and his medical colleagues have treated cancer patients, after surgical removal of the primary tumors, by raising the body temperatures of the patients to about 109° Fahrenheit for an hour, in the hope that the metastases will then be killed or their growth so slowed up as to become harmless. It is not yet decided whether this idea can be described as a practical success, but the provisional work of Von Ardenne is already of great significance in a field where hopes of conventional chemotherapy have been dimmed but might be brightened by a combination with extreme or moderate hypothermia.

A third application is as follows. According to an estimate by K.H. Bauer of the new Cancer Center in Heidelberg, at least one million of the twenty-five million male inhabitants of West Germany will die of cancer of the respiratory tract; still more will die from other inducers of cancer. When one considers that cancer is a permanent menace, one realizes that cancer has become one of the most dangerous menaces in the history of medicine.

Many experts agree that one could prevent about 80% of all cancers in man, if one could keep away the known carcinogens from the normal body cells. The prevention of cancer might involve no great expenses, and especially would require little further research to bring about cancer prevention in up to 80%.

Why does it happen that in spite of all this so little is done towards the prevention of cancer? The answer has always been that one does not know what cancer or the prime cause of cancer is, and that one cannot prevent something that is not known.

But nobody today can say that one does not know what cancer and its prime cause is. On the contrary, there is no disease whose prime cause is better known, so that today ignorance is no longer an excuse that one cannot do more about prevention.

That the prevention of cancer will come there is no doubt, for man wishes to survive. But how long prevention will be avoided depends on how long the prophets of

agnosticism will succeed in inhibiting the application of scientific knowledge in the cancer field. In the meantime, millions of men and women must die of cancer unnecessarily.

Literature to Preface of First Edition:

1. Otto Warburg, A.W. Geissler and S. Lorenz: Uber die letzte Ursache und die entfernten Ursachen des Krebses. 17. Mosbacher Kolioquium, April 1966. Verlag Springer, Heidelberg 1966.
2. Any book on vitamins, such as Th. Bersin. Biochemie der Vitamine. Akad. Verlags.-Ges. Frankfurt, 1966
3. Ernest L. Wynder, Sven Hultberg, Folke Jacobsson and Irwin J. Bross, Environmental Factors in Cancer. Cancer, Vol. 10, 470, 2057.

Literature to Preface of Second Edition:

1. 1) Willstaeter, Wieland and Euler, Lectures on enzymes at the centenary of the Gesellschaft Deutscher Naturforscher.

Berichte der Deutschen Chemischen Gesellschaft, 55, 3583, 1922. The 3 lectures of the 3 famous chemists show that in the year 1922 the action of all enzymes was still a mystery. No active group of any enzyme was known then.

2. Otto Warburg, Biochem. Zeitschrift, 152, 479, 1924.

3. Otto Warburg, Heavy Metals as prosthetic groups of enzymes, Clarendon Press, Oxford 1949.

4. Otto Warburg, Wasserstoffubertragende Fermente, Verlag Werner Sanger, Berlin, 1948.

5. Dean Burk, 1941. On the specificity of glycolysis in malignan Liver tumors as compared with homologous adult or growing liver tissues. In Symposium of Respiratory Enzymes, Univ, of Wisconsin Press, pp. 235-245.1942.

6. Otto Warburg und F. Kubowitz, Biochem. Zeitschrift, 189, 242, 1927; H. Goldblatt und G. Cameron, J. Exper. Med. 97, 525, 1953.

7. Otto Warburg, 17. Mosbacher Kolioquium, April 1966. Verlag Springer, Heidelberg, 1966.

8. Otto Warburg, K. Gawehn, A.W. Geissler, D. Kayser and S. Lorenz, Klinische Wochenschrift 43,289,1965.

9. Otto Warburg, Oxygen, The Creator of Differentiation, Biochemical Energetics, Academic Press, New York, 1966.

10. Otto Warburg, New Methods of Cell Physiology, Georg Thieme, Stuttgart and Interscience Publishers, New York, 1962.

Note by Dean Burk:

This article was adapted from a lecture originally delivered by Otto Warburg at the 1966 annual meeting of Nobelists at Lindau, Germany. Otto Warburg won the Nobel Prize in Medicine in 1931 for his discovery of the oxygen transferring enzyme of cell respiration, and was voted a second Nobel Prize in 1944 for his discovery of the hydrogen transferring enzymes.

Many universities, like Harvard, Oxford, Heidelberg have offered him honorary degrees. He is a Foreign member of the Royal Society of London, a Knight of the Order of Merit founded by Frederick the Great, and was awarded the Great Cross with Star and Shoulder ribbon of the Bundesrepublik. His main interests are Chemistry and Physics of Life. In both fields no scientist has been more successful.

SCIENTIFIC INQUIRY, THE SOMATIDIAN THEORY and AIDS

Presented by Gaston Naessens

to the international Symposium **AIDS: A Different View**

Amsterdam, The Netherlands, 14-16 May, 1992 (trans, from the French by Christopher Bird)

(Scientists sharing presentations at this forum also included, Dr. Peter Duesberg, Dr. Luc Montanier, Dr. Root-Bernstein, Dietmar Schildwaechter, M.D., Ph.D. to name a few.)

I would first like to thank those who have organized this symposium for having afforded me the opportunity to address you all. I am greatly honored to be able to present a portion of my work to so learned an assembly.

I also wish to thank Mr. Christopher Bird for the unstinting support he has brought to a cause that I have heart-feltedly pursued for so many years, as well as for suggestions he has made that demonstrate all his concern for my well-being.

I should like to begin this brief discussion by stressing that the 20th Century scientific mind, in its consideration of the human body mainly as a machine, has been largely occupied with what it could make understandable through physical and chemical analysis. while often neglecting the fact that this same body is an ensemble of structures so intricate as to completely defy human imagination.

As the great scientist Thomas Alva Edison said: **"Until a human being can create a single blade of grass, nature can only laugh at our pseudo-scientific knowledge** Through our modern analytic procedures we understand only an infinitesimal part of the phenomena taking place, each second, within the intimacy of our cells."

Moreover, rather that rejecting out of hand what we do not understand, we should keep an open mind by never forgetting that what nature, in her wisdom, had elaborated over millions of years goes far beyond our intellectual understanding. Man creates nothing!

It is only due to his observational talent, and to his intuition, that he succeeds in using the vital forces gifted him to improve and shape the world he lives in. Nothing in science takes concrete shape that is not the result of patient and industrious research to try to penetrate to the very heart of the mystery of life.

Fundamental research is necessarily a long and persevering task made up of multiple observations and results as satisfying as they are repeatable. And only a discussion of their consequences reflects an attitude of any value toward them. This is an inflexible law for anyone purporting to serve scientific truth.

If one is adept in the experimental method, one has nothing to fear, for insofar as any idea is valid, one continues to develop it; when it is erroneous, experiments serve to rectify it. In all scientific domains, humanity owes its most important progress to the analytic method.

Physicians have made their inventory of the human body as astronomers have made theirs for the cosmos and the physicists and chemists their own for that matter. In so doing, physicians have isolated each bodily organ and separately classified each disease.

At the end of a long analysis they have found, on the one hand, the cell and on the other, the microbe. Technical progress made in the manufacture of laboratory instruments has kept them moving along the track.

New methodologies and devices have led to increasingly profound knowledge of the smallest parts of the human body and have given us a more realistic view of its afflictions.

The humoral theory, an ancient doctrine in medicine, allowed that it was the fluids of the body that permitted disease its traffic. In the mid-18th century, Morgani held that the seat of various maladies lay in specific organs, such as the liver, kidneys, brain, etc. But with the advent of the analytic method, it was shown that the cell was the real locus of an ailment.

In the mid-19th century, the German, Rudolph Virchow, made fundamental discoveries about the life of a cell. He compared the human body to a nation of which each cell was a citizen. Thus, illness came to be seen as a civil war in the heart of that nation.

According to the eminent scientist, no general disease states existed, only afflictions of individual organs and cells, it therefore was no longer necessary to consider the whole ensemble of the organism; it sufficed to consider only its-injured parts. For a whole century, research into the cause of disease was limited to local modifications in tissues.

The idea that general disturbances (excess, emotions, stress) could bring about local anatomical changes began to reappear only in our day. This view has become the foundation for psychophysiology, the importance of which continues to grow. It extends to interest in the linkage, or linkages, that tie the whole of the body to its parts. Only with discoveries by modern endocrinology did it manifest anew.

To recall these facts is not to minimize the merits of the laboratory era which is one of the most brilliant accomplishments in the history of medicine. It is rather to underscore the fact that the analytic method became fruitful only when, after having descended from the whole to its parts, in search of understanding, it climbed back from those parts to the whole, in search of therapeutic action.

Under influence of the analytic method, pharmacopoeia has long ignored the unity of the organism. It has placed its trust in, and its accent on, the selective action of medicinals by establishing a wholly artificial link between the chemistry of inert matter and the chemistry of life.

When, in biology and physiology, one goes from laboratory theory to the realities of daily life, one often has to restate old questions in entirely new terms not only because the parameters requiring integration are so numerous but also because life is apparently something which cannot be reduced to set equations.

For thirty years, the fire power of medicinal drugs has increased by leaps and bounds. Doctors have had at their disposal an arsenal capable of virtually blitzkrieging disease. One only need take the case of antibiotics.

These remedies can bring a halt in just a few days to microbial invasion against which organisms, even with medical assistance, formerly took several weeks to effectively react, if they did not, in fact, succumb to them.

It was believed that the triumph of the new drugs put an end to many medical problems and, never for a moment was it suspected that organisms might simultaneously undergo side effects or that microbial strains might develop resistance to antibiotics.

Their therapeutic value seemed so incontrovertible that little care was taken to examine their inconveniences. Today, the gamut of medicinals available to doctors is so extensive that practically no microorganism can resist them. Yet all the problems of infectious or viral pathology have by no means been resolved.

The microbe's relation to the milieu of its culture, that is to say the body of its host, stands as the principal question to be posed with respect to all organic maladies,

Lately, a new important current in medical research has come on the scene to point up the individuality in each and every patient. The difficulties, or failures, encountered with grafts of living organs or tissues bear witness to the fact that each one of us is profoundly different in makeup from his or her neighbor. Renewed study of the blood returns to define individuality through a formula as personal to any of us as our fingerprints.

If we attentively study the master work Antoine Bechamp has bequeathed us, we shall understand that it is possible to proceed down brand-new roads of research, even if they are not recognized by scientific orthodoxy.

In this domain, it has unfortunately been forgotten that the prime act of experimental medicine is one of persevering observation freed from preconceived ideas, the only basis on which real discovery can depend.

For my part, I do not pretend to have a hold on any all-encompassing truth but, by following in the footsteps of so many research predecessors, I am trying to open the door a little wider to a research approach based on methodical and well-founded observations of certain fundamental biological elements.

A fundamental biological concept always blazes a trail into a land of multiple domains. It is not a fact itself that constitutes a discovery but the new ideas which flow from it. in manifesting one's ideas one must remain free and resilient and unblocked by fear of contradiction of one's theories.

It is by providing hard evidence, in the blood, for- an elementary particle which I have christened the *somatid*, and through my observation of its cycle, that I have been allowed to establish the bases for a new biological conception I have called the somatidian theory.

In 1904, at a conference on AIDS held at Hunter College in New York City, I for the first time had the opportunity to present video-cassette footage, and a series of slides, that illustrated my observations relating to the controversial aspects of this syndrome in light of the somatidian theory.

In 1990, an ever-increasing demand about this theory, and its applications, spurred me to reply to many questions by my organizing a symposium in Quebec which attracted some 200 participants, scientists and biomedical-medical researchers from Canada, thirty-one of the fifty United States and seven foreign countries. At the symposium, I was able to show a second video-cassette entitled: "Somatidian Orthobiology."

Now, in 1992, I have the great pleasure to present to this distinguished audience a third video cassette in which I have attempted to condense, explain and illustrate my view-point with respect to AIDS as seen in the light of my somatidian theory.

I dare to hope that the information it contains will contribute to the advancement of AIDS research.

CONVENTIONAL OPTIONS

Standard Anti-Biotic treatments of cancer

The following excerpts represent the position and progress of F.D.A. approved oncology in both' determining the causes of and providing present day therapies for cancer. They are not intended to encompass the entirety of options but are offered as a requirement of our Institutional Review Board and as a pre-requisite for prudent decisions based upon full disclosure and informed consent.

The following passages have been reproduced *verbatim from the American Medical Association Drug Evaluations*, Fifth Edition, prepared by the A.M.A. Division of Drugs in Cooperation with the American Society for Clinical Pharmacology and Therapeutics, April 1993; from the *Physician's Desk Reference*, 1994 Edition and from *Cancer Control Journal.*, Vol. 5, No. 3/4, 5/6 pp. 61-98.

"Although great efforts have been made in cancer research and major developments have occurred in molecular and cellular biology, many fundamental questions remain unanswered and the etiology and pathogenesis of the basic neoplastic process are still unknown.

"All cancers are malignant tumors characterized by an unlimited growth potential and an ability to expand locally by invasion into surrounding tissues and systemically by metastasis to distant sites in the body." *A.M.A. Drug Evaluations*, 1993, p. 1481.

"The goal of cancer chemotherapy is to achieve selective toxicity against malignant tumor cells and to spare normal host cells." *Ibid.* p. 1482

"Because of the lack of readily exploitable biochemical differences between cancer and normal cells, the cytotoxic (cell destroying) nature of most antineoplastic drugs, and the necessity for optimum dosing for the best response, most anticancer drugs have low therapeutic indices and produce cytotoxic effects in normal cells." *Ibid* p. 1509.

"A variety of antineoplastic drugs, but particularly the alkylating agents, depress spermatogenesis and can cause sterility. Most antineoplastic drugs suppress cellular and humoral immunity. Immunosuppression often does not persist for long periods after treatment is discontinued and is a lesser problem when intermittent scheduling is employed.

"However, since cell-mediated immunity appears to be an important host defense mechanism against the tumor, and the immuno-compromised patient is more susceptible to infection, immuno-suppression is certainly an undesirable toxicity." *Ibid** p. 1510.

"Many of the commonly employed antineoplastic drugs are mutagenic as well as teratogenic and some, including procarbazine hcl and the alkylating agents, are clearly carcinogenic in animals.

"An increase in the frequency of secondary malignancies, particularly acute leukemia, in patients treated for Hodgkin's disease, multiple myeloma, ovarian cancer, and possibly some other cancers have been documented.

The risk of secondary malignancies, which may not appear for many years after successful chemotherapy, must be considered in weighing benefits versus risks for any new therapy." *Ibid* p. 1511.

Cancer Chemotherapy

Antineoplastic Agents

(**neoplasm-any** new and abnormal growth,

Dorland's Illustrated Medical Dictionary, 27th Edition)

Other than the hormonal agents, there are four groups of antineoplastic (anticancer) agents-alkylating, antimetabolites, antibiotics and alkaloids, and miscellaneous. They inhibit malignant cells to varying degrees during various parts of the cell cycle, that is, they are poisonous, depending on their toxicity to interfere with the growth of the malignant cells.

Unfortunately, in comparison to other classes of drugs, these chemotherapeutic drugs are distinguished by a low therapeutic index, reflecting their relative inability to discriminate effectively between normal and malignant, cells. Thus, they are cytotoxic rather than tumoricidal. The premise for their use is that normal cells have a greater capability for repair than most malignant cells.

The effect of these anticancer agents on the life cycle of the cell varies. The pharmacology of antineoplastic agents is complex, but generally they may be divided into two groups: (1) the cycle-specific agents, which destroy cells in any phase of the cell cycle although they preferentially kill in one phase compared to another. (2) the **phase-specific agents**, which kill cells selectively in one phase of the cell cycle and therefore have little if any effect on nonproliferating cells even at a relatively high dose.

1. **The cycle-specific agents** include the **alkylating agents**, such as cyclophosphamide CYTOXAN and HN2 MUSTARGEN, a nitrogen mustard, most **antineoplastic antibiotics**, and procarbazine hydrochloride **MATULANE**, a miscellaneous agent.

2. The **phase-specific agents**, which usually attack the S-DNA synthesis phase of the life-cycle of the cell, include most **antimetabolites** (agents that inhibit the utilization of products of metabolism), the **vinca alkaloids**, and possibly the antibiotic bleomycin BLENOXANE. CCJ, Vol. 5, no. 3/4, 5/6, pp.62-63.

corticosteroids

The corticosteroids stimulate the bone marrow and are used for the treatment of the leukemias and lymphomas. Long-term use of corticosteroids may cause swelling, with a Cushingoid blowed-up appearance, endocrine abnormalities, hypertension, musculoskeletal problems, peptic ulceration, acute pancreatitis, infections, euphoria, insomnia, psychosis, atrophy, acne, and excessive growth of hair. They also may inhibit growth in children, *ibid.* p.66.

Prednisone; classified as an *adrenal corticosteroid*

delayed major toxicity, bone marrow depression (primarily leukopenia, thrombocytopenia); alopecia; skin hyper-pigmentation, pulmonary fibrosis (uncommon) indications: acute and chronic lymphocytic leukemia; Hodgkin's and non-Hodgkin's lymphomas; multiple myeloma; breast carcinoma. *AMA Drug Evaluations*

hormones

The effect of hormones on the body is quite different from the other antineoplastic agents, as their action does not depend on toxicity, but rather on their regulatory mechanism.

Little is known of the progressive histological changes that may occur following hormone therapy. Hormones are palliative; that is, they provide temporary regression of the malignancy, not permanent. CCJ, *op. cit. p. 65*

Diethylstilbestroi (DES); classified as *estrogen*;

acute major toxicity, occasional nausea

delayed major toxicity fluid retention, hypercalcemia; feminization; uterine bleeding increased frequency of vascular accidents (especially at high doses); vaginal carcinoma in offspring of pregnant women given drug

indications: prostatic and breast carcinomas (postmenopausal women).

Several reports suggest there is an association between intrauterine exposure to female sex hormones and congenital anomalies, including congenital heart defects and limb- reduction defects.

warnings: "Diethylstilbestrol should not be used for any purpose during pregnancy. Its use may cause severe harm to the fetus." *PDR* 48th Edition, 1994 p. 1200.

megace; (megestrol acetate tablets), a progestin.

Clinical pharmacology, While the precise mechanism by which Megace produces its antineoplastic effects against endometrial carcinoma is unknown at the present time, inhibition of pituitary gonadotropin production and resultant decrease in estrogen secretions may be factors.

Indications and Usage; Megace is indicated for the palliative treatment of advanced carcinoma of the breast or endometrium (i.e. recurrent, inoperable or metastatic disease). It should not be used in lieu of currently accepted procedures such as surgery, radiation or chemotherapy.

Warnings: Megestrol acetate may cause fetal harm when administered to a pregnant woman.

Precautions: Carcinogenesis, Mutagenesis, and Impairment of Fertility: Administration for up to 7 years of megestrol acetate to female docs is associated with an increased incidence of both benign and malignant tumors of the breast. Comparable studies in rats and in monkeys are not associated with an increased incidence of tumors. The relationship of the dog tumors to humans is unknown but should be considered in assessing the benefit-to-risk ratio when prescribing Megace and in surveillance of patients on therapy. *Ibid.*, p. 659.

alkyiating agents

The alkylating agents are highly toxic, no doubt killing the cell by cross-linking DNA. These agents differentiate very little between malignant and normal tissue. Most antineoplastic antibiotics, such as ADRIAMYCIN, inhibit DNA and/or RNA, which carries out DNA instructions synthesis. *CCJ, op cit.*, p. 62.

Cytoxan; (cyclophosphamide), a synthetic, antineoplastic and progestational drug.

Clinical pharmacology; cytoxan is biotransformed principally in the liver to active alkylating metabolites by a mixed function microsomal oxidase system.

These metabolites interfere with the growth of susceptible rapidly proliferating malignant cells. The mechanism of action is thought to involve cross-linking of tumor cell DNA.

Indication and usage: 1) malignant lymphomas, Hodgkin's disease, lymphocytic lymphoma, mixed-cell type lymphoma, histiocytic lymphoma, Burkitt's lymphoma 2) Multiple myeloma 3) Leukemias 4) Mycosis fungoides 5) Neuroblastoma 6) Adenocarcinoma of the ovary 7) Retinoblastoma 8) Carcinoma of the breast.

Warnings: carcinogenesis, mutagenesis, impairment of fertility; second malignancies have developed in some patients treated with cyclophosphamide used alone or in association with other antineoplastic drugs and/or modalities. Cyclophosphamide can cause fetal harm when administered to a pregnant woman and such abnormalities have been reported following cyclophosphamide therapy in pregnant women. Infections; treatment with cyclophosphamide may cause significant suppression of immune responses. Serious, sometimes fatal, infections may develop in severely immunosuppressed patients.

Precautions: General; special attention to the possible development of toxicity should be exercised in patients being treated with cyclophosphamide if any of the following conditions are present: 1. leukopenia, 2. thrombocytopenia, 3. tumor infiltration of bone marrow, 4. previous X-Ray therapy, 5. Previous therapy with other cytotoxic agents, 6. Impaired hepatic function, 7. Impaired renal function. PDR, *op.cit.* p. 654.

antimetabolite

Antimetabolites are antagonists of folic acid, purine, or pyrimidine. For example, METHOTREXATE, inhibits the reduction of folic acid and interferes with tissue-cell reproduction. Vitamin preparations containing folic acid interfere with the effect of this drug. THIOGUANINE and PURINETHANOL block purine metabolism, and FLUOROURACIL pyrimide metabolism. CCJ, op. cit. p. 62.

methotrexate; cell cycle specificity S-phase specific but self-limiting;

acute major toxicity, mild nausea and vomiting; diarrhea; acute hypersensitivity reactions; delayed major toxicity bone marrow depression (leukopenia, anemia, thrombocytopenia); oral and gastrointestinal ulceration; renal tubular necrosis; hepatic fibrosis, pneumonitis; osteoporosis;

Indications: choriocarcinoma; acute lymphocytic leukemia; non-Hodgkin's and Burkitt's lymphomas; osteogenic sarcoma; rhabdomyosarcoma; testicular cancer; head and neck, breast, lung, cervical, ovarian and bladder carcinomas; medulloblastoma; mycosis fungoides.

Warning. Methotrexate must be used only by physicians experienced in antimetaboiite chemotherapy. Because of the possibility of serious toxic reactions, the patient should be fully informed by the physician of the risks involved and should be under his constant supervision. Deaths have been reported with the use of methotrexate in the treatment of malignancy, psoriasis and rheumatoid arthritis. PDR, op.cit., p. 1072

Fluorouracil, (5FU)

Clinical pharmacology; Fluorouracil interferes with the synthesis of DNA and to a lesser extent inhibits the formation of RNA.

Indications and usage; Fluorouracil is effective in the palliative management of carcinoma of the colon, rectum, breast, stomach and pancreas.

Contraindicated for patients in a poor nutritional state, those with depressed bone marrow function, those with potentially serious infections or those with a known sensitivity to Fluorouracil.

Warnings; The daily dose of Fluorouracil is not to exceed 500MG. It is recommended that patients be hospitalized during their first course of treatment.

Precautions: Fluorouracil is a highly toxic drug with a narrow margin of safety.

Adverse reactions: stomatitis, esophagopharyngitis, diarrhea, anorexia, nausea and emesis are commonly seen during therapy. Leukopenia usually follows every course of adequate therapy with Fluorouracil. Other adverse reactions are to the blood, heart, intestinal system, brain, skin, eyes, mental stability and miscellaneous such as thrombophlebitis, epistaxis and loss of nails. *PDR., op.cit.*, p. 1924.

anti-biotics

Most antineoplastic antibiotics, such as ADRIAMYCIN, inhibit DNA and/or ANA (ribonucleic acid, the messenger that carries out the DNA's instructions) synthesis by binding to or complexing with DNA. CCJ, op. cit, p. 63.

Adriamycin; Doxorubicin Hydrochloride cell cycle specificity nonspecific; S-phase probably most sensitive;

acute major toxicity, nausea and vomiting; diarrhea; red urine (not hematuria); local irritant; transient EKG changes

delayed major toxicity, bone marrow depression (leukopenia, thrombocytopenia, anemia); cardiac toxicity including irreversible congestive heart failure (total cumulative dose should not exceed 550 mg/M2); alopecia; stomatitis; fever and chills;

'*indications:* acute myelogenous and acute lymphocytic leukemia; Hodgkin's and non- Hodgkin's lymphomas, multiple myeloma; testicular cancer; breast, lung, gastric, pancreatic, carcinomas; osteogenic, Ewing's and soft tissue sarcomas; rhabdomyosarcoma; Wilm's tumor; neuroblastoma. *PDR, op.cit.*, p. 458.

miscellaneous agents

The miscellaneous agents are not classified because they either differ in their function from the other groups or their action is not known. Most of these agents are investigational.*CCJ, op. cit.* p. 63

platinol (cisplatin);

Warning: cumulative renal toxicity associated with Platinol is severe. Other major dose- related toxicities are myelosuppression, nausea, and vomiting. Ototoxicity, which may be more pronounced in children, and is manifested by tinnitus [ringing or buzzing in the ears], and/or loss of high frequency hearing and occasional deafness, is significant. Anaphylactic-like reactions [life-threatening respiratory distress followed by vascular collapse] to Platinol have been reported. Facial edema, bronchoconstriction, tachycardia, and hypotension may occur within minutes of Platinol administration. Epinephrine, corticosteroids, and antihistamines have been effectively employed to alleviate symptoms.

Indications; metastatic testicular tumors..., metastatic ovarian tumors.... advanced bladder cancer.

Contraindications: Platinoi is contraindicated in patients with preexisting renal impairment. Platino! should not be employed in myelosuppressed patients, or patients with hearing impairment. *PDR. op. cit.* p. 666.

carboplatin, (paraplatin)

Warning: Bone marrow suppression is dose related and may be severe, resulting in infection and/or bleeding. Anemia may be cumulative and may require transfusion support. Vomiting is another frequent drug-related side-effect. Anaphylactic-like reactions have been reported and may occur within minutes of Paraplatin administration. *PDR, op. cit.*, p. 662.

The vinca alkaloids, vinblastine and vincristine, are the salts of an alkaloid extracted from the periwinkle plant. They appear to act as mitotic inhibitors by blocking division of the cell. *CCJ, op. cit.*, p. 63.

Vincristin (Oncovin)

Uses: Hodgkin's disease, lymphosarcoma, reticulum cell sarcoma, rhabdomyosarcoma, neuroblastoma, Wilms' tumor.

Pharmaceutical toxicity:

Contraindications: there are no contraindications but careful attention should be given to those conditions listed under Warning and Precautions.

Warning: Since reproductive studies have not been performed in animals, there is insufficient information as to whether this drug may affect fertility in men and women or have teratogenic or other adverse effects on the fetus.

Adverse Reactions: in general, adverse reactions are reversible and are related to dosage. The most common adverse reaction is hair loss; the most troublesome are neuromuscular in original. Other adverse reactions that have been reported are abdominal cramps, ataxia, foot drop, weight loss, fever, cranial nerve manifestations, paresthesia and numbness of the digits, polyuria, dysuria, oral ulceration, headache, vomiting and diarrhea. *PDR, op. cit.*, p. 1268.

Important toxicities to individual organs

and the antineoplastic drugs most frequently implicated are as follows:

sMn-bleomycin (very common and includes hyper-pigmentation, induration, erythema, vesicles, bullae)

lung—bleomycin (usual dose limiting toxicity; most often pneumonitis, but fatal pulmonary fibrosis can occur), busulfan and chloroethyl nitrosoureas (pulmonary fibrosis) and *methotrexate* (pneumonitis)

heart-doxorubicin [Adriamycin] and *daunorubicin* (cumulative toxicity that limits total dose to 550 mg/M2; ranges from transient

EKG changes to cardiomyopathy with irreversible congestive heart failure)

liver-mercaptopurine, thioguanine, and sex steroids (cholestatic jaundice), asparaginase (fatty metamorphosis) and methotrexate (fibrosis and cirrhosis with prolonged use)

pancreas-asparaginase (hyperglycemia, hemorrhagic pancreatitis) and *streptozocin* (hyperglycemia)

Kidney-c/sp/at/n (usual dose-limiting toxicity; acute renal tubular necrosis), *streptozocin* (usual dose-limiting toxicity; ranges from proteinuria to renal tubular atrophy), *cloroethy! nitrosoureas* and *mitomycin* (delayed onset nephrotoxicity that can progress to renal failure). *A M. A. Drug Evaluations*, 1993, p. 1510.

Chemotherapy, like much of the technology of radiation therapy, had its origins in war, in this case in the development of poison gases during World War II. Toward the end of the Italian campaign, Axis forces detonated a U.S. ship loaded with poison mustard gas that was anchored in Naples harbor.

Some observant doctors noted that many of the American sailors died of bone marrow poisoning (anemia and lack of white blood cells, which are made in the marrow). It was quickly reasoned that nitrogen mustard, a toxic component of the gas, might treat leukemia, which is a blood cancer characterized by excessive production of immature white cells.

Shortly after the war, Dr. Sidney Farber of Boston is said to have extended the lives of several leukemia patients by administering methotrexate. *CCJ, op. cit.* p. 118.

RADIOTHERAPY

Radiotherapy, like surgery, is a localized treatment for cancer. The primary goal is to destroy the malignant cells of the tumor. Irradiation is generally used for tumors not accessible or appropriate for surgery.

It is prudent to assume that whenever the body tissue is irradiated, even with a minimal dose, there is damage to the tissue. According to Dr. Brass of Roswell Park Memorial Institute in Buffalo, New York, it takes very little radiation to impair the defense mechanism of the human body and we cannot even assume that dosages under 5 rads are harmless, as something we can tolerate.

Before submitting to radiotherapy for the treatment of cancer, it is certainly wise to become aware of the potential risks of this method of treatment. Not only are some people more severely affected by irradiation than others, but many organs of the body are more vulnerable to damage than others, causing death or morbidity. The effects of irradiation may be far worse than the discomfort or dangers caused by the malignancy.

The organs most severely injured by radiotherapy are the brain, heart, lungs, spinal cord, stomach, liver, intestine, kidney, fetus and bone marrow. Radiation lesions are fatal or result in severe morbidity to 1 to 5% of patients on a minimal dose; 25 to 50% of patients on maximal dose who have received radiation to these organs.

The realm of radioactive agents includes a wide variety of radiation sources. Intense highly localized deposition of ionizing radiation is achieved by the interstitial implantation or intracavitary placement of capsules, needles, tubes, threads, and other devices containing natural or artificial radioactive isotopes.

Four of the radioactive isotopes used for therapeutic treatment of cancer include Au Gold- grain, Sodium Iodide 1 131, Sodium Phosphate P 32, and Cobalt 60.

There may be increased risks when radiotherapy and chemotherapy are combined. Certain cancer drugs markedly enhance radiation injury when given either before during, or after irradiation, and this interaction can cause severe morbidity.

The potential of second malignancies following both chemotherapy and radiotherapy is particularly high. Bender and Young cite a study that states that patients who received intensive chemotherapy and radiotherapy had a 29-fold increase of either modality alone.

The immunological system, especially the lymph nodes, bone marrow components, spleen, and thymus are extremely sensitive to irradiation. When the immunological system is damaged, the body becomes less resistant to infections, and subsequent metabolic therapy may be less effective.

Also, genetic damage by radiation to the younger generation who produce offspring may affect their children, leading to leukemia. According to a study presented by Dr. Bross, the incidence of leukemia among one-to-four-year old children of parents who had radiation previous to their birth is about four times of those whose parents had no radiation.

Whether radiotherapy is effective or not depends on whether the radiation used was appropriate for that particular malignancy, whether the quality of life is unduly affected by the therapy, and whether the malignancy is really under control.

One of the important factors in the administration of radiotherapy is the equipment. Contemporary radiotherapy is carried out with Y rays as well as X rays. X or roentgen rays are the electro-magnetic ionizing radiation produced by man-made machines, whereas y rays emanate from naturally occurring or artificially produced radioactive elements such as radium or cobalt 60. In the past only the very low energy beams of kilovoltage X rays, appropriate for lesions of limited depth and palliation, were used.

Today, very high energy X rays are provided by megavoltage devices such as linear electron accelerators and beatrons, which have properties essentially indistinguishable from those of the radioactive cobalt, used for deep-seated radiation.

With ordinary X-ray therapy, two or three times as much radiation is required for cells that are low in oxygen. Fast neutron therapy, which is administered only at certain cancer centers, differs from other radiation therapies in that it is less dependent on an adequate supply of oxygen in the tumor, which makes it appropriate for radiation of large tumors. These tumors have a tendency to outgrow their blood supply, with a consequent development of viable tumor cells low in oxygen.

The fear that late effects would be excessive has held back the use of fast neutron therapy. Such information appears scanty, but the effect of fast neutron therapy on the rapidly proliferating cells responsible for early radiation damage and the slowly dividing cells for late radiation damage is similar to that of X rays. However, the repair of sub-lethal (slightly less than death of organ) damage is less or slower after neutron therapy. Because of this factor, retreatment could be hazardous.

These new radiotherapy devices are very expensive and still investigational, without being proved by medical experience. Such large investments would tend to make them a permanent part of the cancer therapy program, though there may develop contradictions to their use, particularly because of late toxicities.

CCJ, op cit, pp. 91-99.

The following is excerpted verbatim from the U.S. Code of Federal Regulations which contains "the general and permanent laws of the United States in force on January 3, 1989?

The Code of Federal Regulations (CFR), title 21

defines the general standards for the composition, operation, and responsibility of an IRB that reviews clinical investigations regulated by the Food and Drug Administration under Sections 505(i), 507(d) and 520(g) of the act, as well as clinical investigations that support applications for research or marketing permits for products regulated by the Food and Drug Administration including food and color additives, drugs for human use, biological products for human use and electronic products.

Compliance with this part is intended to protect the rights and welfare of human subjects involved in such investigations.

(b) References in this part to regulatory sections of the Code of Federal Regulations are to Chapter I of title 21 CFR Ch. 1 (4-1-91 Edition), unless otherwise noted. CFR part 56.102 Definitions.

The Act as used in this part means the Federal Food, Drug, and Cosmetic Act, as amended (secs.902, 52 Stat. 1040 et seq. as amended (21 U.S.C. 321*392).

Application for research or marketing permit and information regarding a substance submitted as part of the proceedings for establishing that a substance is generally recognized as safe for use which results or may reasonably be expected to result, directly or indirectly, in its becoming a component or otherwise affecting the characteristics of any food, described in part 170.35.

(6) An Investigational new drug application, described in part 312 of this chapter.

(9) Data and information regarding an over©the©counter drug for human used submitted as part of the procedures for classifying such drugs as generally recognized as sage and effective and not misbranded, described in part 330.

(11) An application fora biological product license, described in part 601.

(12) Data and information regarding a biological product submitted as part of the procedures for determining that licensed biological products are safe and effective and not misbranded, as described in part 601.1

Clinical investigation means any experiment that involves a test article and one or more human subjects, and either must meet the requirements for submission to the Food and Drug Administration under section 505 (i), 50 (d), or 520 (g) of the act, or need not meet the requirements for prior submission to the F.D.A. under these sections of the act, but results of which are intended to be later submitted to, or held for inspection by, the F.D.A. as part of an application for a research or marketing permit.

Emergency use means the use of a test article on a human subject in a life-threatening situation in which no standard acceptable treatment is available, and in which there is no sufficient time to obtain IRB approval. Institution means any public or private entity or agency (including Federal, State, and other agencies).

The term facility as used in this section 520(g) of the act is deemed to be synonymous with the term institution(g) Institutional Review Board (IRB) means any board, committee, or other group formally designated by an institution to review, to approve the initiation of, and to conduct periodic review of, biomedical research involving human subjects. The primary purpose of such review is to assure the protection of the rights and welfare of the human subjects. The term has the same meaning as the phrase institutional review committee has used in section 520 (g) of the act.

(h)lnvestigator means an individual who actually conducts a clinical investigation (i.e., under whose immediate direction the test article is administered or dispensed to, or used involving, a subject) or, in the event of an investigation conducted by a team of individuals, is the responsible leader of that team.(i) Minimal risk means that the risks of harm anticipated in the proposed research are not greater, considering probability and magnitude, than those ordinarily encountered in daily life or during the performance of routine physical or psychological examinations or tests.

Sponsor means a person or other entity that initiates a clinical investigation, but that does not actually conduct the investigation, I.E., the test article is administered or dispensed to, or used involving, a subject under the immediate direction of another individual. A person other than an individual (e.g., a corporation or agency) that uses one or more of its own employees to conduct an investigation that it has initiated is considered to be a sponsor (not sponsor investigator), and the employees are considered to be investigators.

Sponsor investigator means an individual who both initiates and actually conducts, alone or with others, a clinical investigation, i.e., under whose immediate direction the test article is administered or dispensed to, or used involving, a subject. The term does not include any person other than an individual, e.g., it does not include a corporation or agency. The obligations of a sponsor or investigator under this part include both those of a sponsor and those of an investigator.

Test article means any drug for human use, biological product for human use, medical device for human use, human food additive, color additive, electronic product, or any other article subject to regulation under the act or under sections 351 or 354 or 360F of the Public Health Service Act. (46FR 8975, Jan.27, 1981, as amended at 54 FR 9038, Mar. 3, 1989] Part 56.103 Circumstances in which IRB review is required.

(a)Except as provided in Parts 56.104 and 56.105, any clinical investigation which must meet the requirements of prior submission (as required in 312, 812, and 013) to the Food and Drug Administration shall not be initiated unless that investigation has been reviewed by, and remains subject to continuing review by, an IRB meeting the requirements of this part.(b)

Except as provided in parts 56.104 and 56.105, the Food and Drug Administration may decide not to consider in support of an application for a research or marketing permit any data or information that has been derived form a clinical investigation that has not been approved by, and that was not subject to initial and continuing review by, and IRB meeting the requirements of this part.

The determination that a clinical investigation may not be considered in support of an application for research or marketing permit does not, however, relieve the applicant for such a permit of an obligation under any other applicable regulations to submit the results of an investigation to the Food and Drug Administration, (c) Compliance with these regulations will in no way render inapplicable pertinent Federal, State, or local laws or regulations. 46 FR 8975, Jan. 27 1981 ;46 FR 14340, Feb. 27, 1901H Part 56,104

Exemptions from IRB requirement

The following categories of clinical investigations are exempt from the requirements of this part of IRB review:

(a) Any investigation which commenced before July 27, 1901 and was subject to requirements for IRB review under FDA regulations before that date, provided that the investigation remains subject to review of an IRB which meets the FDA requirements in effect before July 27, 1981.

(c) Emergency use of a test article, provided that such emergency use is reported to the IRB within five working days. Any subsequent use of the test article at the institution is subject to IRB review. Part 56.105 Waiver of IRB requirement. On the application of a sponsor or sponsor investigator, the Food and Drug Administration may waive any of the requirements contained in these regulations, including the requirements for IRB review, for specific research activities or for classes of research activities, otherwise covered by these regulations. Subpart B -

Organization and Personnel Part 56.107 IRB Membership.

(a)Each IRB shall have at least five members, with varying backgrounds, to promote compete and adequate review of research activities commonly conducted by the institution. The IRB shall be sufficiently qualified through the experience and expertise of its members, and the diversity of the members' backgrounds including consideration of the racial and cultural backgrounds of members and sensitivity to such issues as community attitudes, to promote respect for its advice and counsel in safeguarding the rights and welfare of human subjects.

In addition to possessing the professional competency necessary to review specific research activities, the IRB shall be able to ascertain the acceptability of proposed research in terms of institutional commitments and regulations, applicable law, and standards of professional conduct and practice.

The IRB shall therefore include persons knowledgeable in these areas. If an IRB regularly reviews'research that involves a vulnerable category of subjects, including but not limited to subjects covered by other parts of this chapter

, the IRB should include one or more individuals who are primarily concerned with the welfare of these subjects.

(b)No IRB may consist entirely of men, or entirely of women, or entirely of members of one profession.

(c)Each IRB shall include at least one member whose primary' concerns are in nonscientific areas.

(d)Each IRB shall include at least one member who is not otherwise affiliated with the institution and who is not part of the immediate family of a person who is affiliated with the institution.

(e)No IRB may have a member participate in the IRB's initial or continuing review of any project in which the member has a conflicting interest, except to provide information requested by the IRB.

(f)An IRB may, in its discretion, invite individuals with competence in special areas to assist in the review of complex issues which require expertise beyond or in addition to that available on the IRB. These individuals may not vote with the IRB

Sub part C -IRB Functions and Operations. Part 56.100 IRB functions and operations.

In order to fulfill the requirements of these regulations, each IRB shall:

a. Follow written procedures

1. for conducting its initial and continuing review of research and for reporting its findings and actions to the investigator and the institution,

2. for determining which projects require review more often than annually and which projects need verification from sources other than the investigators that no material changes have occurred since previous IRB review,

3. for insuring prompt reporting to the IRB of changes in research activity,

4. for ensuring that changes in approved research, during the period for which IRB approval has already been given, may not be initiated without IRB review and approval except where necessary to eliminate apparent immediate hazards to the human subjects, and

5. for insuring prompt reporting to the IRB of unanticipated problems involving risks to subjects or others.

b. Except when an expedited review procedure is used (see part 56.110), review proposed research at convened meetings at which a majority of the members of the IRB are present, including at least one member whose primary concerns are in nonscientific areas. In order for the research to be approved, it shall receive the approval of a majority of those members present at the meeting.

c. Be responsible for reporting to the appropriate institutional officials and the Food and Drug Administration any serious or continuing noncompliance by investigators with the requirements and determinations of the IRB.

Part 56.109 IRB review of research,

a. An IRB shall review and have authority to approve, require modifications in (to secure approval), or disapprove all research activities covered by these regulations. (b) An IRB shall require that information given to subjects as part of informed consent is in accordance with Part 50.25. The IRB may require that information, in addition to that specifically mentioned in Part 50.25, be given to the subjects when in the IRB's judgment the information would meaningfully add to the protection of the rights and welfare of subjects.

b. An IRB shall require documentation of informed consent in accordance with Part 50.27, except that the IRB may, for some or all subjects, waive the requirement that the subject or subjects legally authorized representative sign a written consent form if it finds that the research presents no more than minimal risk of harm to subjects and involves no procedures for which written consent is normally required outside the research context. In cases where the documentation requirement is waived, the IRB may require the investigator to provide subjects with a written statement regarding the research.

c. An IRB shall notify investigators and the institution in writing of its decision to approve or disapprove the proposed research activity, or of modifications required to secure IRB approval of the research activity. If the IRB decides to disapprove a research activity, it shall include in its written notification a statement of the reasons for its decision and give the investigator an opportunity to respond in person or in writing.

d. An IRB shall conduct continuing review of research covered by these regulations at intervals appropriate to the degree of risk, but not less that once per year, and shall have authority to observe of have a third party observe the consent process and the research.

Part 56,110 Expedited review procedures for certain kinds of research involving no more than minimal risk, and for minor changes in approved research.

a. The Food and Drug Administration has established, and published in the FEDERAL REGISTER a list of categories of research that may be reviewed by the IRB through an expedited review procedure. The list will be amended, as appropriate, through periodic republication in the FEDERAL REGISTER.

b. An IRB may review some or all of the research appearing on the list through an expedited review procedure, if the research involves no more than minimal risk. The IRB may also use the expedited review procedure to review minor changes in previously approved research during the period for which approval is authorized. Under an expedited review procedure, the review may be carried out by the IRB chairperson or by one or more experienced reviewers designated by the chairperson from among the members of the IRB. In reviewing the research, the reviewers may exercise all of the authorities of the IRB except that the reviewers may not disapprove the research. A research activity may be disapproved only after review in accordance with non-expedited procedures sei forth in Part 56.108(b).

c. Each IRB which uses and expedited review procedure shall adopt a method for keeping all members advised of research proposals which have been approved under the procedure,

d. The Food and Drug Administration may restrict, suspend, or terminate an institution's or IRB's use of the expedited review procedure when necessary to protect the rights of welfare of the subjects.

Part 56.111 Criteria of IRB approval of research.

a. In order to approve research covered by these regulations the IRB shall determine that all of the following requirements are satisfied:

1. Risks to subjects are minimized: (i) By using procedures which are consistent with sound research design and which do not unnecessarily expose subjects to risk, and (ii) whenever appropriate, by using procedures already being performed on the subjects for diagnostic or treatment purposes,

2. Risks to subjects are reasonable in relation to anticipated benefits, if any, to subjects and the importance of the knowledge that may be expected to result. In evaluating risks and benefits, the IRS should consider only those risks and benefits that may result from the research (as distinguished from risks and benefits of therapies that subjects would receive even if not participating in the research). The IRB should not consider possible long Orange effects of applying knowledge gained in the research (for example, the possible effects of the research on public policy) as among those research risks that fall within the purview of its responsibility.

3. Selection of subjects is equitable. In make this assessment, the IRB should take into account the purpose of the research and the setting in which the research will be conducted.

4. Informed consent will be sought from each prospective subject or the subject's legally authorized representative, in accordance with and to the extent required by part 50i i

5. Informed consent will be appropriately documented in accordance with and to the extent required by Part 50.27.

6. Where appropriate, the research plan makes adequate provisions for monitoring the data collected to ensure the safety of subjects.

7. Where appropriate, there are adequate provisions to protect the privacy of the subjects and to maintain the confidentiality of data,

b. Where some or all of the subjects are likely to be vulnerable to coercion or undue influence, such as persons with acute or severe physical or mental illness, or persons who are economically or educationally disadvantaged, appropriate additional safeguards have been included in the study to protect the rights and welfare of these subjects.

Part 56.112 Review by Institution.

Research covered by these regulations that has been approved by an IRB may be subject to further appropriate review and approval or disapproval by officials of the institution. However, those officials may not approve the research if it has not been approved by an IRB.

Part 56.113 Suspension or termination of IRB approval of research.

An IRB shall have authority to suspend or terminate approval of research that is not being conducted in accordance with the IRB's requirements or that has been associated with unexpected serious harm to subjects. Any suspension or termination of approval shall include a statement of the reasons for the IRB's action and shall be reported promptly to the investigator, appropriate institutional officials, and the Food and Drug Administration.

Part 56.114 Cooperative Research

In complying with these regulations, institutions involved in multi-institutional studies may use joint review, reliance upon review of another qualified IRB, or similar arrangements aimed at avoidance of duplication of effort.

Subpart D - Records and Reports Part 56.115 IRB Records

a. An institution, or where appropriate an IRB, shall prepare and maintain adequate documentation of IRB activities, including the following:

1. Copies of all research proposals reviewed, scientific evaluations, ff any, that accompany the proposals, approved sample consent documents, progress reports submitted by investigators, and reports of injuries to subjects,

2. Minutes of IRB meetings which shall be in sufficient detail to show attendance at the meetings; actions taken by the IRB; the vote on these actions including the number of members voting for, against, and abstaining; the basis for requiring changes in or disapproving research; and written summary of the discussion of controverted issues and their resolution.

3. Records of continuing review activities.

4. Copies of all correspondence between the IRB and the investigators.

5. A list of the IRB members identified by name; earned degrees; representative capacity; indications of experience such as board certifications, licenses, etc., sufficient to describe each member's chief anticipated contributions to IRB deliberations; and any employment or other relationship between each member and the institution; for example full-time employee,

part-time employee, a member of a governing panel or board, stockholder, paid or unpaid consultant.

6. Written procedures for the IRB as required by Part 56.108 (a).

7. Statements of significant new findings provided to subjects, as required by Part 50.25.

b. The records required by this regulation shall be retained for at least 3 years after the completion of the research, and the records shall be accessible for inspection and copying by authorized representatives of the Food and Drug Administration at reasonable times and in a reasonable manner.

c. The Food and Drug Administration may refuse to consider a clinical investigation in support of an application for a research or marketing permit if the institution or the IRB that reviewed the investigation refuses to allow an inspection under this section.

Subpart E (c) Administrative Actions for Noncompliance
Part 56,120 Lesser administrative actions.

a. If apparent noncompliance with these regulations in the operation of an IRB is observed by an FDA investigator during an inspection, the inspector will present an oral or written summary of observations to an appropriate representative of the IRB. The Food and Drug Administration may subsequently send a letter describing the noncompliance to the IRB and to the parent institution. The agency will require that the IRB or parent institution respond to this letter within a time period specified by FDA and describe the corrective actions that will be taken by the IRB, the institution or both to achieve compliance with these regulations.

b. On the basis of the IRB's or the institution's response, FDA may schedule a reinspection to confirm the adequacy of corrective actions. In addition, until the IRB or the parent institution takes appropriate corrective action, the agency may:

1. Withhold approval of new studies subject to the requirements of this part that are conducted at the institution or reviewed by the IRB.

2. Direct that no new subjects be added to ongoing studies subject to this part.

3. Terminate ongoing studies subject to this part when doing so would not endanger the subjects; or

4. **When the apparent noncompliance creates a significant threat to the rights and welfare of human subjects, notify relevant State and Federal regulatory agencies and other parties with a direct interest in the agency's action of the deficiencies in the operation of the IRB.**

c. The parent institution is presumed to be responsible for the operation of an IRB, and Food and Drug Administration will ordinarily direct any administrative action under this subpart against the institution. However, depending on the evidence of responsibility for deficiencies, determined during the investigation, the Food and Drug Administration may restrict its administrative actions to the IRB or to a component of the parent institution determined to be responsible for formal designation of the IRB.

Part 56.121 Disqualification of an IRB or an institution

a. Whenever the IRB or the institution has failed to take adequate steps to correct the noncompliance stated in the letter sent by the agency under Part 56.120 (a), and the Commissioner of Food and Drugs determines that this noncompliance may justify the disqualification of the IRB or the parent institution, the Commissioner will institute proceedings in accordance with the requirements for a regulatory hearing set forth in part 16.

b. The Commissioner may disqualify an IRB or the parent institution of the Commissioner determines that:

   1. The IRB has refused or repeatedly failed to comply with any of the regulations set forth in this part, and

   2. The noncompliance adversely affects the rights or welfare of the human subjects in a clinical investigation.

c. If the Commissioner determines that disqualification is appropriate, the Commissioner will issue an order that explains the basis for the determination and that prescribes any actions to be taken with regard to ongoing clinical research conducted under the review of the IRB, The Food and Drug Administration will send notice of the disqualification to the IRB and the parent institution. Other parties with a direct interest, such as sponsors and clinical investigators, may also be sent a notice of the disqualification. In addition, the agency may elect to publish a notice of its action in the FEDERAL REGISTER.

d. The Food and Drug Administration will not approve an application for a research permit for a clinical investigation that is to be under the review of disqualified IRB or that is to be conducted at a disqualified institution, and may refuse to consider support of a marketing permit the data from a clinical investigation that was reviewed by a disqualified IRB as conducted at a disqualified institution unless the IRB or the parent institution is reinstated as provided in Part 56.123.

Part 56.122 Public disclosure of information regarding revocation.

A determination that the Food and Drug Administration has disqualified an institution and the administrative record regarding that determination are disclosable to the public under part Part 56.123

Reinstatement of an IRB or an institution. An IRB or an institution may be reinstated if the Commissioner determines, upon an evaluation of a written submission from the IRB or institution that explains the corrective action that the institution or IRB plans to take, that the IRB or institution has provided adequate assurance that will operate in compliance with the standards set forth in this part. Notification of reinstatement shall be provided to all persons notified under Part 56.121(c).

Part 56.124 Actions alternative or additional to disqualification.

Disqualification of an IRB or of an institution is independent of, and neither in lieu of nor a precondition to, other proceedings or actions authorized by the act. *The Food and Drug Administration may, at any time through the Department of Justice institute any appropriate judicial proceedings (civil or criminal) and any other appropriate regulatory action, in addition to or in lieu of, and before, at the time of, or after, disqualification. The agency may also refer pertinent matters to another Federal, State, or local government agency for any action that agency determines to be appropriate.*

THE UNITED STATES CODE TITLE 21 FOOD AND DRUGS

The Code of Federal Regulations (CFR) contains a codification of Documents of General Applicability and future effect and is Published by the Office of the Federal Register National Archives and Records Administration.

(CFR) Part 56 Institutional Review Boards

(CFR) 50.27

Subpart B-Informed Consent of Human Subjects

a. Except as provided in 56.109(c), informed consent shall be documented by the use of a written consent form approved by the IRB and signed by the subject or the subject's legally authorized representative, A copy shall be given to the person signing the form.

b. Except as provided in 56/109(c), the consent form may be either of the following:

1. A written consent document that embodies the elements of informed consent required by 50.25. This form may be read to the subject or the subject's legally authorized representative, but, in any event, the investigator shall give either the subject

or the representative adequate opportunity to read it before it is signed.

2. A short form written consent document stating that the elements of informed consent required by 50.25 have been presented orally to the subject or the subject's legally authorized representative. When this method is used, there shall be a witness to the oral presentation.

NEW DRUGS

[**Ed. Note:** Camphor has been used in traditional medicine for over 5,000 years. Congress has granted powers to a department of the executive branch of Government known as Health and Human Services, which is responsible for the agency known as the Food and Drug Administration. This Agency is mandated to regulate the sale and use of all Food and Drug substances.]

THE UNITED STATES CODE OF FEDERAL REGULATIONS,

Title 21, Food and Drugs contains these general and evolving regulations,]

CFR 21 Part 310.100 Subpart A * General Provisions

(g)New Drug Substance means any substance that when used in the manufacture, processing, or packing of a drug to be a new drug, but does not include intermediaries used in the synthesis of such substance,

(h) The newness of a drug may arise by reason (among other reasons) of:

1. The newness for drug use of any substance which composes such drug, in whole or in part, whether it be an active substance or a menstruum, excipient, carrier, coating, or other component.

2. The newness for a drug use of a combination of two or more substances, none of which is a new drug.

3. The newness for drug use of the proportion of a substance in a combination, even though such combination containing such substance in other proportion is not a new drug.

4. The newness of use of such drug in diagnosing, curing, mitigating, treating, or preventing a disease, or to affect a structure or function of the body, even though such drug is not a new drug when used in another disease or to affect another structure or function of the body.

5. (5) The newness of a dosage, or method or duration of administration or application, or other condition of use prescribed, recommended, or suggested in the labeling of such drug, even though such drug when used in other dosage, or other method or duration of administration or application, or different condition, is not a new drug,

(j) The term sponsor means the person or agency who assumes responsibility for an investigation of a new drug, including responsibility for compliance with applicable provisions of the act and regulations.

The "sponsor" may be an individual, partnership, corporation, or Government agency and may be a manufacturer, scientific institution, or an investigator regularly and lawfully engaged in the investigation of new drugs.

Part 360.j (g) (l)Exemptions for devices for investigational use

(1) It is the purpose of this subsection to encourage, to the extent consistent with the protection of the public health and safety and with ethical standards, the discovery and development of useful devices intended for human use and to that end to maintain optimum freedom for scientific investigators in their pursuit of that purpose.

BIBLIOGRAPHY

Atkins, Robert C., M.D., Dr. Atkin's New Diet Revolution.

The American Health Empire: Power, Profits and Politics, a Report from the Health Policy Advisory Center (Health- PAC),

The American Medical Association, Drug Evaluations, 5th Edition, April 1983, prepared by the AMA Division of Drugs, in Cooperation with the American Society for Clinical Pharmacology and Therapeutics.

Balch, James, M.D and Phyllis A., C.N.C., Prescription for Nutritional Healing: A Practical A-Z reference to Drug* Free remedies using vitamins, minerals, herbs & food Supplements.

Bird, Christopher; The Persecution and Trial of GASTON NAESSENS: The True Story of the Efforts to Suppress an Alternative Treatment for Cancer, AIDS, and Other Immunologically Based Diseases., (319 pages), H J. Kramer, Inc., Tiburon, CA, 1990, second edition 1991.

Brecher, Harold and Arline, Forty Something Forever: A consumer's guide to chelation therapy.

Captan, Arthur L., If I were a rich man could I buy a pancreas? and other essays on the ethics of health care. Indiana University Press, Bloomington and Indianapolis, 1992.

Carter, James P., M.D., D.P.H. Racketeering in Medicine: The Suppression of Alternatives, Hampton Roads Publishing Company, Inc., Norfolk, VA.

Coulter, Harris L., Ph.D., The Controlled Clinical Trial, Center for Empirical Medicine, Washington, D.C., 1991.

Coulter, Harris L., Ph.D., A Divided Legacy: A History of the Schism in Medical Thought: Vol, L the Patterns Emerge: Hippocrates to Paracelsus. (560 pages) Weehawken Book Company, Washington, D.C., 1975.

Cranton, Elmer; Bypassing Bypass: The New Techniques of Chelation Therapy, by Hampton Roads Publishing Company, Norfolk, VA.

Fink, John M., Third Opinion, An International Directory to Alternative Therapy Centers for the Treatment and Prevention of Cancer and Other Degenerative Diseases, Avery Publishing.

GAO/PEMD 90-15 FDA, Drug Review; Post approval risks 1976-85.

Gerson, Max, M.D., <u>A Cancer Therapy: Results of Fifty Cases</u>.

Gray, Bradford H., <u>The Profit Motive and Patient Care, the Changing Accountability of Doctors and Hospitals</u>, Harvard University Press, Cambridge, MA; London, 1991,

Greenberg. Selig, <u>The Quality of Mercy, Atheneum</u>, New York 1971.

Gregory, Scott, O.M.D., <u>A Holistic Protocol for the Immune System</u>,

Guthrie, Randolph H., M.D., <u>The Truth about Breast Implants, forward by Betty Rollin, author of First You Cry</u>, John Wiley & Sons, Inc., 1994.

Heimlich,. Jane, <u>What your Doctor Won't Tell You</u>, by Harper/Collins Publishers.

Martin, E.W. et al: <u>Hazards of Medication</u>, Toronto: J.B. Lippincott, Co. 1971.

McCabe, Ed, <u>O2ygen Therapies: A New Way of Approaching Disease</u>.

Mendelsohn, Robert S.t M.D. <u>Confessions of a Medical Heretic</u>, Contemporary Books, 1979.

Moss, Ralph, *The Cancer Industry: The Classic Expose on the Cancer Establishment*, Paragon House, NYC, NY 1989,

Mullins, Eustace, *<u>Murder by Injection</u>,*

Naessens, Gaston, "Somatidian Orthobiology", VHS video showing live footage of the somatid cycle, the somatoscope and method of injection. * "Aids and the Somatidian Theory."

New England Journal of Medicine, Vol 314, No, 19, "Progress Against Cancer/ by John C. Bailar III and Elaine M. Smith, May 8, 1986.

The New England Journal of Medicine, Special Article, Unconventional Medicine the United States, Prevalence, Costs and Patterns of Use., David M. Eisenberg, MD., Ronald C. Kessler, Ph.D,, Cindy Foster, M.P.H., Frances E. Norlock, M.P.H., David R. Calkins, M.D,, M.P.P and Thomas L. Delbanco, M.D., January 20, 1993.

Page, Benjamin L, Who Gets What From the Government, Univ, of California Press, Berkeley, Los Angeles, London, 1983.

Payer, Lynn; Disease Mongers, John Wiley & Sons, Inc., New York, Toronto, 1992.

"The Rights Retained by the People, The History and Meaning of the Ninth Amendment." A publication of the Center for Constitutional Studies of the Cato Institute, Edited by Randy E. Barnett.

Strecker, Robert, M.D. The Strecker Memorandum on AIDS, Eagle Rock, CA.

Tompkins, Peter and Bird, Christopher, Secrets of the Soil: New Age Solutions for Restoring our Planet, Perennial Library, Harper & Row Publishers, 1989.

United States General Accounting Office, Washington, DC 20548, Program Evaluation and Methodology Division, letter reference B-235044, April 26, 1990.

Vithoulkas, George; *A New Model of Health and Disease, Suggesting and Explanation for the Explosion of Aids, Cancer, Asthma, Candida, Epilepsy, Alzheimer's, Tuberculosis, Schizophrenia, MS, Allergic conditions, Rheumatoid Arthritis and Chronic Fatigue,* published by Health and Habitat and North Atlantic Books, 199k

Warren, Tom, Beating Alzheimer's: A Step Towards Unlocking the Mysteries of Brain Diseases, Avery Publishing.

West, Stanley, M.D. and Dranov, Paula; The Hysterectomy Hoax, Doubleday, 1994.

Wohl, Stanley, M.D. The Medical Industrial *Complex*, Harmony Books, New York, 1984.

LEGAL REFERENCES

Amsler v. Verrilli, 119 A.D. 2d 786, 501 N.Y.S. 2d 411 (2d Dep't 1986).

Blacks Law Dictionary, Fifth Edition, Copyright 1891, 1979, by West Publishing Company, pg. 289.

Bovard, James, Lost Rights, The Destruction of American Liberty, 1994, Scholarly and Reference Division, St. Martins Press, Inc., pg. 333.

B.Y.U. Journal of Pubiic Law, Vol 6, No. 603, "Oksanen v. Page Memorial Hospital: The Fourth Circuit's Antitrust Analysis for Peer Review Actions Under the Sherman Act/ by Grant L. Kratz, Boston.

The Constitution of the United States of America.

DePaul Law Review, Vol, 39, "The Future of Hospital Peer Review Committees in the Antitrust Arena," by Susan Capra, Chicago, Spring 1990,

The Douglas Opinions, Edited by Vern Countryman, Random House, 1977.

Duquesne Law Review, Vol 28. "Antitrust Liability in the Context of Medical Peer Review: The implications of Patrick v. Burget and the Health Care Quality Improvement Act of 1986/, by Jennifer Otto, Pittsburgh, Spring 1990.

"The Economist," February 4th, 1995.

895 Federal Reporter, 2d Series, "Wilk v. American Medical Association/ United States Court of Appeals, Seventh Circuit; argued Dec 1, 1988, decided Feb. 7, 1990; Rehearing and Rehearing En Banc Denied in No. 87-2672, April 25,1990.

micro cycle, stages of the Somatid Cycle 1-3. microbial globular, a microscopic bacterium filled with gloves of material. Micron, one millionth of a meter, or one thousandth of a millimeter, the ratio between an inch and a micron is the same as the Empire State Building at 1,470 feet high to a firefly.

milieu, surroundings, environment.

mitosis, the process by which the body grows and replaces cells, consisting of a complex of various processes, by means of which the two daughter nuclei normally receive identical complements of the number of chromosomes characteristic of the somatic cells of the species,

motile, having spontaneous but not conscious or volitional movement.

motility, the ability to move spontaneously.

myco, a combining form meaning related to fungus.

mycoplasma, a taxonomic name given a genus, of the family Mycoplasmataciae, including the pleuropneumonia-like organisms (PPLO) and separated into 15 species on the basis of source, glucose fermentation, and growth on agar media. (An agar medium is a special medium that is indigestible by bacteria.)

mycelial forms, (mycelium) a mass of threadlike strands, filaments found on fungi,

mycelium, active, a mass of threadlike strands, filaments with motile particles inside.

myelin, any one of a certain group of lipid substances found in various normal and pathologic tissues and different from fats in being doubly refractive.

myelinic, pertaining to the nature of the myelin.

necrosis: the sum of the morphological changes indicative of cell death and caused by the progressive degradative action of enzymes.

neoplasia, the progressive multiplication of cells under conditions that would not elicit, or would cause cessation of, multiplication of normal cells.

neuroblastoma: sarcoma of nervous system origin.

numerical aperture, deals with the magnification factor of the optics of the microscope rather than the resolution factor of the material in the specimen under view.

osmosis, the passage of pure solvent from a solution of lesser to one of greater solute concentration when the two solutions are separated by a membrane which selectively prevents the passage of solute molecules, but is permeable to the solvent.

osmotic, pertaining to or of the nature of osmosis.

pancreatitis: acute or chronic inflammation of the pancreas; acute p., a form characterized by sudden onset of abdominal pain, nausea, and vomiting, acute hemorrhagic p., a condition due to autolysis of pancreatic tissue caused by the escape of enzymes into its substance.

phagocytic, the process by which some cells in the body eat or consume small living things and various wastes by an ingestion or engulfing action.

pleomorphic, the ability of an organism to alter its living form during growth similar to a tadpole evolving into a frog; e.g. the various forms of the Somatid Cycle display the Somatid's pleomorphic abilities.

phlegmasical reticulum, having to do with phlegm or heat inflammation, the area of clotting resembling a cluster when viewed through the dark field microscope.

phlegmatic, characterized by an excess of the supposed humor called phlegm; hence heavy, dull, and apathetic.

pulmonary fibrosis: formation of fibrous tissue in the lung.

pneumonitis: inflammation of the lungs.

proteinuria: the presence of an excess of serum proteins in the urine.

thrombocytopenia: decrease in the number of blood platelets.

resolution, in addition to the magnification factor or numerical aperture of microscopes, the work of Royal Raymond Rife and Gaston Naessens reveals additional areas in which microscopes can be enhanced in order to reveal new structure and new information in the specimens being studies. One need only to think of a field full of fireflies in the daylight. As one gazes out across the field, the presence of thousands of fireflies, with the exception of an occasional undefined insect taking to flight in the breeze, goes virtually unnoticed. At a distance and under these lighting conditions it is next to impossible to resolve the nature of the insect observed or others resting in the plant tops. Increasing magnification will not assist the observer in locating, isolating or differentiating the insects to any single firefly for examination. As the evening approaches and under proper lighting conditions, the task of resolving fireflies by their flashes of light becomes easier. In the darkness of the night, thousands upon thousands of fireflies are easily targeted and individually resolved. Magnification can now be affected to reveal new structure.

Under dark field examination it is the various materials making up the structure of the cells or microorganism under view that appear to glow and emit light of their own into viewing eyepieces. The microorganisms emit their own light on a dark field back drop rather than a reflection of light off of the surface of the object being viewed.

For the past 46 years Gaston Naessens has evolved this process a step further by introducing various selective frequencies of light, by electronic means, into the dark field. Fine forms and delicate structures hitherto unresolved by normal reflective means resonate and become visible in the plasma and the cells. It is these particles that are changing the way we perceive the biology of the body and its systems. Gaston Naessens has opened the door to new vistas relating to our understanding of the true nature of the body's degenerative processes.

Additional scientific information is now being added to a holistic view of health and our growing data base of biological knowledge.

sarcoma: a tumor made up of a substance like the embryonic connective tissue; tissue composed of closely packed cells embedded in a fibrillar or homogeneous substance, often highly malignant.

teratogenic, producing physical defects (monstrosities) in offspring in *utero*.

Informed Consent and Petition Constitutional and Human Rights

The Declaration of Helsinki Human Rights Accord, of which the United States is a signatory, adopted by the 18th World Medical Assembly, Helsinki, Finland, 1964 and reaffirmed again in 1989 contains the following statement:

"In the treatment of a sick person, the doctor must be free to use a new therapeutic measure, if in his judgment it offers hope of saving life, re-establishing health or alleviating suffering."

California and Universal Bill of Rights for treatment by any modality accepted or experimental.

You have been asked, or have yourself asked, to participate as a subject in an experimental clinical procedure. Before you decide whether you want to participate in the experimental procedure, you have a right to:

1. Be informed of the nature and purpose of the treatment whether experimental or conventional therapy.

2. Be given an explanation of the procedures to be followed in the medical experiment, and any drug or device to be utilized.

3. Be given a description of any attendant discomforts and risks reasonably to be expected from your participation in the experiment;

4. Be given an explanation of any benefits reasonably to be expected from your participation in the experiment;

5. Be given a disclosure of any appropriate alternative procedures, drugs or devices that might be advantageous to you and their relative risks and benefits;

6. Be informed of the avenues of medical treatment, if any, available to you after the experimental procedure if complications should arise;

7. Be given an opportunity to ask any questions concerning the medical experiment or the procedures involved;

8. Be instructed that consent to participate in the experimental procedure may be withdrawn at any time and that you may discontinue participation in the medical experiment without prejudice;

9. Be given a copy of this form and the signed and dated written consent form.
10. Be given the opportunity to decide to consent or not to consent to the medical experiment without the intervention of any element of force, fraud, deceit, duress, coercion or undue influence on your decision.

I have of my own free will chose to participate in this project in an endeavor to restore my health and exercise my rights to Life, Liberty and the Pursuit of Happiness as set forth in the Declaration of Independence.

Title, purpose and procedures

Through the United States' endorsement of the Helsinki Accord and my assertion of my Constitutional rights under the Ninth Amendment, I understand that, as a citizen of the United States of America, I am entitled to seek treatment for myself according to my own best judgment with any medication available internationally even if it is not available to me in my own country.

I understand that this project, entails the application of a camphor compound, TRIMETHYLBICYCLONITR AMINOHEPTANE CL, also known as 714X, in the treatment of CANCER and other viral, immuno-deficient and degenerative diseases such as MS, C F S, A L S, LUPUS, Rheumatoid Arthritis and AIDS so that it may be approved for general usage.

I understand I will be expected to participate for an undetermined time of at least six months for life threatening situations according to the protocol established by Gaston Naessens and the Chief Investigator, the length of individual treatment to be determined by the severity of my case in concurrence with the Chief Investigator.

The procedure for usage has been clearly explained to me as a series of intra-lymphatic injections in the right inguinal lymph node, which may be supplemented by daily or replaced by twice daily nebulization, if injections are not possible.

RISKS:

As part of this program, I understand that I may choose to have my blood drawn for a nominal fee which may be reimbursable by my insurance company, for the purpose of tests at the time of or prior to the administration of the drug and at times throughout the treatment procedure in order to monitor the effects of treatment and progression or regression of the disease.

I understand that there are no other known or reported risks from those having used 714X on human subjects. The only known side-effects are a possible burning sensation from the camphor or pain from the injection which generally subsides quickly, or possible formation of a small bruise or slight numbness at the site of injection.

BENEFITS:

I understand that the benefits may be the amelioration or complete remission of the condition for which I am being treated by a process which serves to stabilize the immune function. Because this substance is banned in the United States by Federal Bureaucracy this study is considered experimental according to the rules and regulations of the FDA. We are required to state the following:

I am aware that there are no guarantees of success and it is possible that the desired benefits or that unforeseen complications arising out of my illness or from previous treatment, complications including worsening of my condition or death may occur.

RESEARCH RELATED INJURY:

If research-related injury is sustained in the course of participation in the study I understand that appropriate medical attention is my responsibility in consultation with my primary physician. Should I sustain injury as a result of this study I understand no compensation is provided.

ALTERNATIVE TREATMENTS:

In the case of cancer, I understand that other therapies are available to me including radiation, surgery and chemotherapy.

COSTAND PARTICIPATION REIMBURSEMENT:

To date most Insurance Carriers do not cover costs of unapproved medicine. I understand there will be a standard cost for the 714X.

Consultation with co-investigators and fees for project-related professional service between myself and my chosen professional, physician or medical personnel will be determined on an individual basis and are not the province of this I.R.B. There will be no reimbursement for participation.

MEDICAL RECORDS:

I may choose to release my medical records pertaining to the condition for which I am being treated with 714X and those obtained in the course of this research project to the I. R. B. I understand that these documents will be accessible to parties involved in the production and development of the research project. I understand that these records will be used, without reference to my name, for purposes of substantiating the findings of the project.

LIABILITY RELEASE:

Signing this consent document does not waive my rights nor does it release the investigators or sponsors from their responsibilities.

SIGNIFICANT NEW FINDINGS:

I have been told that should my disease become worse, should side-effects become severe, should new scientific developments occur that indicate the treatment is not in my best interest, or should I agree with my physician that this treatment is no longer in my best interest, then the treatment would be stopped and further treatment would be discussed.

PARTICIPANTS RIGHTS:

Participation is voluntary and I will suffer no penalty or loss of benefits to which I am otherwise entitled by refusal to participate or by withdrawing my consent to participate at any time.

If I have any question or comments relating to this research project, I understand I can contact my primary physician and/or the Sponsors of this project.

FOR THE RECORD

There is no substitute for personal, direct communication and success of treatment is in great measure based on this foundation. However, a background of information can be helpful both to place events in your own mind and give us a general picture of your history and condition.

To better serve you and the requirements of scientific documentation, we would appreciate if you fill out the following client questionnaire. This is purely voluntary and the information contained will be used only for internal purposes for your benefit and anonymously for the benefit of the IRB.

1. Name
2. Address:
3. Phone: Fax:
4. Date and full descriptive name of original diagnosis (i.e. type of cancer, cell type or histology, location, stage, primary,

metastatic, etc.) for which you are treating yourself at this time.

5. Date of recurrences, including metastatic diagnoses, if any.

6. Prior treatment:

A. SURGERY: description and dates.

Were you informed of the risks and side effects? What were you told after surgery?

What were the results of this treatment?

1. immediate:
2. long term:

B. CHEMOTHERAPY: names, dosages and dates of treatment. Were you informed of the risks and specific side effects?

What were you told concerning the results of this treatment?

What were the results of this treatment?

1. immediate:
2. long term:

C. RADIATION: areas, length per dose, intensity, and dates.

Were you informed of the risks and side effects? What were you told concerning the results of this treatment?

What were the results of this treatment?

1. immediate
2. long term

D. OTHER ALLOPATHIC TREATMENTS: Le., Taxol, tamoxifen, antibiotics such as Adriamycin, vancomycin hcl.

Were you informed of the risks and side effects?

What were you told concerning the results of this treatment?

What were the results of this treatment?

1. immediate:
2. long term:

E. NON-ALLOPATHIC TREATMENT: (this includes all treatments that do NOT use surgical or pharmaceutical intervention), names, dates.

What were you told concerning the results of this treatment? What were the results of this treatment?

1. immediate:
2. long-term:
3. Were you informed of any other therapies available worldwide?
4. Was your treatment covered by medical insurance?
5. What was the cost of your entire treatment? Charged to insurance:

Personal expense:

1. If you have no clinical diagnosis, what are the symptoms causing you to seek treatment?

2. Are you being treated for or aware of any other disease? Which ones?

3. What medications or supplementations are you taking? List all by name and dosage.

4. How do you rate your present state of health?

5. Are you aware that it is possible to restore health?

6. To what origin or origins do you trace your present state of disease, i.e. mental or emotional distress, physical trauma, extraordinary exposure to any of the following chemical agents: pesticides, silicone, benzene, radiation, fluoride, mercury, etc.

7. Do you have mercury amalgam fillings in your mouth?

8. What is the history of chronic and/or degenerative disease in your family?

9. Do you have copies of all your medical records? If not, you may wish to request them for your personal files and for possible future documentation and testimony by Writers and Research, Inc

10. Do you have an interest in expressing your experience and views on the socio/political front communicating with representatives, interviews with the media, participation in legal action for change?

11. We frequently receive requests by potential or active patrons to speak with someone familiar with this treatment. Are you interested in offering assistance to other patrons in the future?

Please feel free to add any comments on a separate sheet.

I have read the questionnaire, the contents of this document and of the consent form and have listened to the verbal explanation. My questions concerning this study have been answered to my satisfaction. I hereby give voluntary consent to participate in this study (or for my child to participate in this study).

I have read and been given a copy of this four (4) page consent form.

I have elected to treat myself for the following condition/disease: please print:

Name of patron (please print) Date

Nota Bene-. The Board may approve by oral consent procedure which does not include or which alters some or all of the above elements or may waive the requirement to obtain consent provided the Board finds and documents that: The research involves no more than minimal risk to the patron.

The waiver or alternation will not adversely affect the rights and welfare of the patron. The research could not practicably be carried out without the waiver or alteration. Whenever appropriate, the subjects will be provided with additional pertinent information during and or after participation.

PLEASE RETURN YOUR CONSENT FORM

THE RIGHT TO TRY ACT

One Hundred Fifteenth Congress
of the United States of America

AT THE SECOND SESSION

Begun and held at the City of Washington on Wednesday, the third day of January, two thousand and eighteen

An Act

To authorize the use of unapproved medical products by patients diagnosed with

a terminal illness in accordance with State law, and for other purposes.

Be it enacted by the Senate and House of Representatives of the United States of America in Congress assembled,

SECTION 1. SHORT TITLE.

This Act may be cited as the "Trickett Wendler, Frank Mongiello, Jordan McLinn, and Matthew Bellina Right to Try Act of 2017".

SEC. 2. USE OF UNAPPROVED INVESTIGATIONAL DRUGS BY PATIENTS

DIAGNOSED WITH A TERMINAL ILLNESS.

(a) IN GENERAL. —Chapter V of the Federal Food, Drug, and Cosmetic Act is amended by inserting after section 561A (21 U.S.C. 360bbb–0) the following:

"SEC. 561B. INVESTIGATIONAL DRUGS FOR USE BY ELIGIBLE PATIENTS.

"(a) DEFINITIONS. —For purposes of this section—

"(1) the term 'eligible patient' means a patient—

"(A) who has been diagnosed with a life-threatening disease or condition (as defined in section 312.81 of title 21, Code of Federal Regulations (or any successor regulations));

"(B) who has exhausted approved treatment options and is unable to participate in a clinical trial involving the eligible investigational drug, as certified by a physician, who—

"(i) is in good standing with the physician's licensing organization or board; and

"(ii) will not be compensated directly by the manufacturer for so certifying; and

"(C) who has provided to the treating physician written informed consent regarding the eligible investigational drug, or, as applicable, on whose behalf a legally authorized representative of the patient has provided such consent;

"(2) the term 'eligible investigational drug' means an investigational drug (as such term is used in section 561)—

"(A) for which a Phase 1 clinical trial has been completed;

"(B) that has not been approved or licensed for any use under section 505 of this Act or section 351 of the Public Health Service Act;

S. 204—2

"(C)(i) for which an application has been filed under section 505(b) of this Act or section 351(a) of the Public Health Service Act; or

"(ii) that is under investigation in a clinical trial that—

"(I) is intended to form the primary basis of a claim of effectiveness in support of approval or licensure under section 505 of this Act or section 351 of the Public Health Service Act; and

"(II) is the subject of an active investigational new drug application under section 505(i) of this Act or section 351(a)(3) of the Public Health Service Act, as applicable; and

"(D) the active development or production of which is ongoing and has not been discontinued by the manufacturer or placed on clinical hold under section 505(i); and

"(3) the term 'phase 1 trial' means a phase 1 clinical investigation of a drug as described in section 312.21 of title 21, Code of Federal Regulations (or any successor regulations).

"(b) EXEMPTIONS.—Eligible investigational drugs provided to eligible patients in compliance with this section are exempt from sections 502(f), 503(b)(4), 505(a), and 505(i) of this Act, section 351(a) of the Public Health Service Act, and parts 50, 56, and 312 of title 21, Code of Federal Regulations (or any successor

regulations), provided that the sponsor of such eligible investigational
drug or any person who manufactures, distributes, prescribes, dispenses, introduces or delivers for introduction into interstate commerce, or provides to an eligible patient an eligible investigational
drug pursuant to this section is in compliance with the applicable requirements set forth in sections 312.6, 312.7, and 312.8(d)(1) of title 21, Code of Federal Regulations (or any successor regulations) that apply to investigational drugs.

"(c) USE OF CLINICAL OUTCOMES.—

"(1) IN GENERAL.—Notwithstanding any other provision of this Act, the Public Health Service Act, or any other provision of Federal law, the Secretary may not use a clinical outcome associated with the use of an eligible investigational drug pursuant to this section to delay or adversely affect the review or approval of such drug under section 505 of this Act or section 351 of the Public Health Service Act unless—

"(A) the Secretary makes a determination, in accordance with paragraph (2), that use of such clinical outcome is critical to determining the safety of the eligible investigational drug; or

"(B) the sponsor requests use of such outcomes.

"(2) LIMITATION. —If the Secretary makes a determination under paragraph (1)(A), the Secretary shall provide written notice of such determination to the sponsor, including a public health justification for such determination, and such notice shall be made part of the administrative record. Such determination shall not be delegated below the director of the agency center that is charged with the premarket review of the eligible investigational drug.

"(d) REPORTING. —

"(1) IN GENERAL. —The manufacturer or sponsor of an eligible investigational drug shall submit to the Secretary an annual summary of any use of such drug under this section. The summary shall include the number of doses supplied, the

S. 204—3

number of patients treated, the uses for which the drug was made available, and any known serious adverse events. The Secretary shall specify by regulation the deadline of submission of such annual summary and may amend section 312.33 of title 21, Code of Federal Regulations (or any successor regulations) to require the submission of such annual summary in conjunction with the annual report for an applicable investigational new drug application for such drug.

"(2) POSTING OF INFORMATION. —The Secretary shall post an annual summary report of the use of this section on the internet website of the Food and Drug Administration, including the number of drugs for which clinical outcomes associated with the use of an eligible investigational drug pursuant to this section was—

"(A) used in accordance with subsection (c)(1)(A);

"(B) used in accordance with subsection (c)(1)(B); and

"(C) not used in the review of an application under section 505 of this Act or section 351 of the Public Health Service Act.".

(b) NO LIABILITY. —

(1) ALLEGED ACTS OR OMISSIONS. —With respect to any alleged act or omission with respect to an eligible investigational drug provided to an eligible patient pursuant to section 561B of the Federal Food, Drug, and Cosmetic Act and in compliance with such section, no liability in a cause of action shall lie against—

(A) a sponsor or manufacturer; or

(B) a prescriber, dispenser, or other individual entity (other than a sponsor or manufacturer), unless the relevant conduct constitutes reckless or willful misconduct, gross negligence, or an intentional tort under any applicable State law.

(2) DETERMINATION NOT TO PROVIDE DRUG. —No liability shall lie against a sponsor manufacturer, prescriber, dispenser or other individual entity for its determination not to provide access to an eligible investigational drug under section 561B of the Federal Food, Drug, and Cosmetic Act.

(3) LIMITATION. —Except as set forth in paragraphs (1) and (2), nothing in this section shall be construed to modify or otherwise affect the right of any person to bring a private action under any State or Federal product liability, tort, consumer protection, or warranty law.

SEC. 3. SENSE OF THE SENATE.

It is the sense of the Senate that section 561B of the Federal Food, Drug, and Cosmetic Act, as added by section 2—

(1) does not establish a new entitlement or modify an existing entitlement, or otherwise establish a positive right to any party or individual;

(2) does not establish any new mandates, directives, or additional regulations;

(3) only expands the scope of individual liberty and agency among patients, in limited circumstances;

(4) is consistent with, and will act as an alternative pathway alongside, existing expanded access policies of the Food and Drug Administration;

S. 204—4

(5) will not, and cannot, create a cure or effective therapy where none exists;

(6) recognizes that the eligible terminally ill patient population often consists of those patients with the highest risk of mortality, and use of experimental treatments under the criteria and procedure described in such section 561A involves an informed assumption of risk; and

(7) establishes national standards and rules by which investigational drugs may be provided to terminally ill patients.

Speaker of the House of Representatives.

Vice President of the United States and

President of the Senate.

DETERMINATION

There is no chance, no destiny, no fate,
Can circumvent or hinder or control
The firm resolve of a determined soul.
Gifts count for nothing; will alone is great;
All things give way before it,
soon or late.

What obstacle can stay the mighty force
Of the sea-seeking river in
its course,
Or cause the ascending orb
of day to wait?

Each well-born soul must win what
it deserves.
Let the fool prate of luck. The fortunate
Is he whose earnest purpose never swerves,
Whose slightest action or
inaction serves

The one great aim, Why,
even Death stands still,
And waits an hour sometimes
for such a will.

ELLA WHEELER WILCOX

Made in the USA
Lexington, KY
08 November 2019